Wound Healing

Edited by Muhammad Ahmad

Published in London, United Kingdom

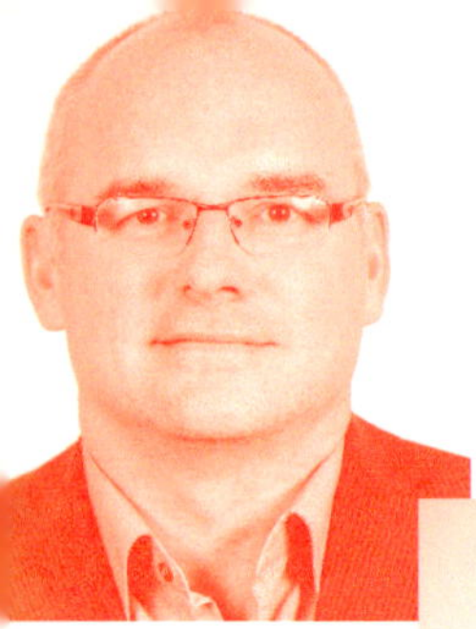
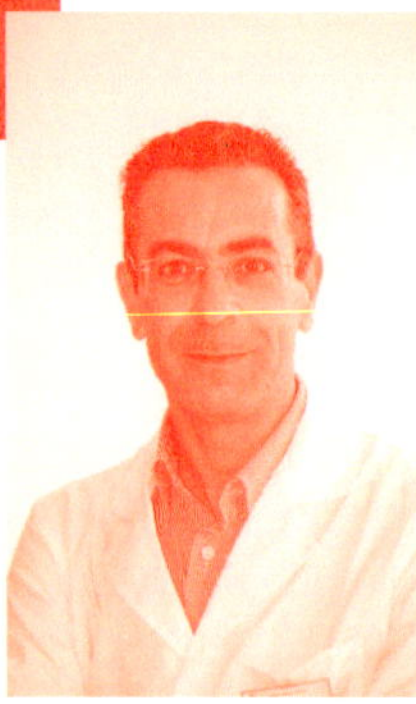
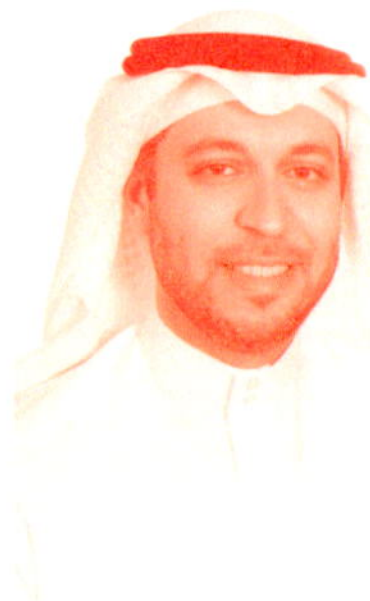
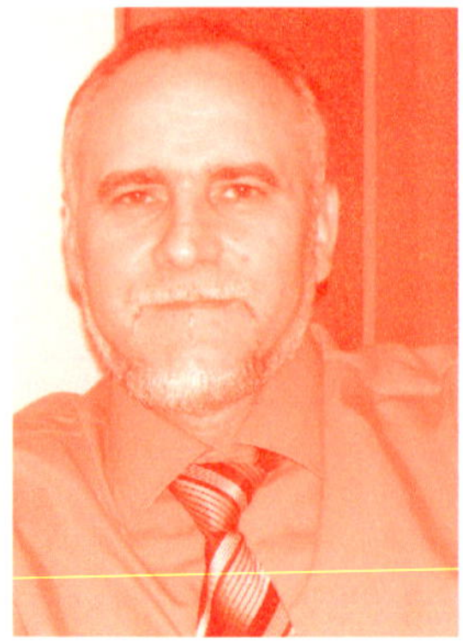
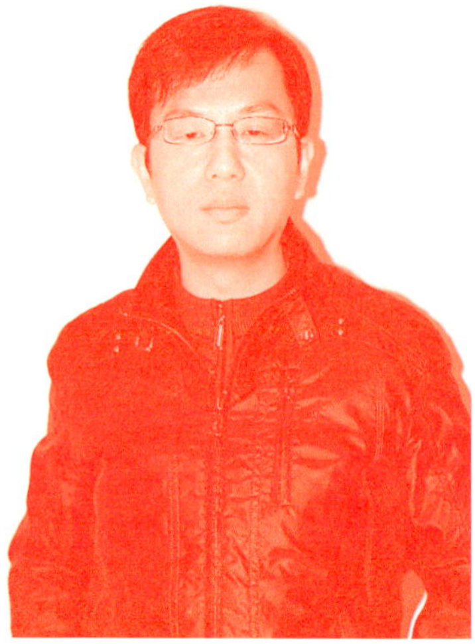
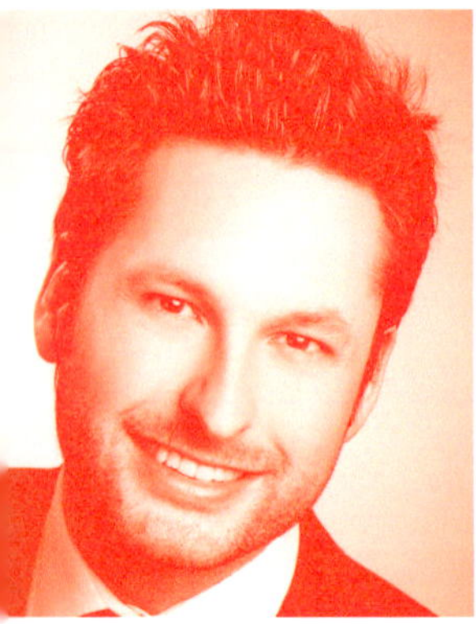
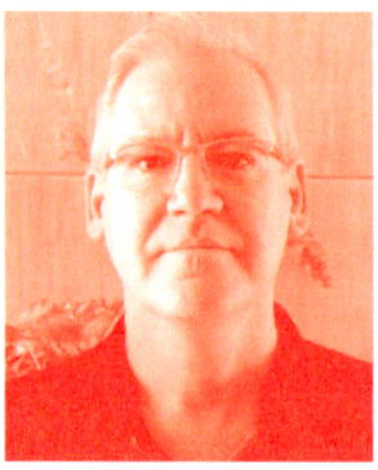

IntechOpen

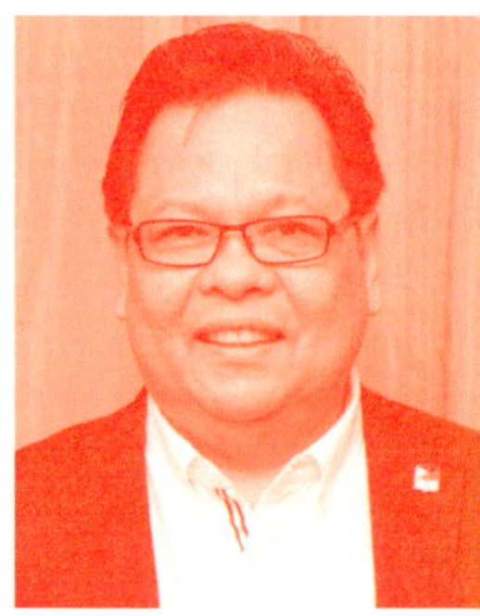
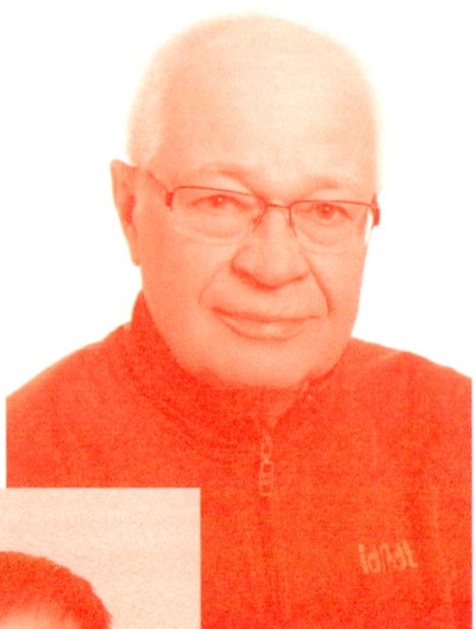
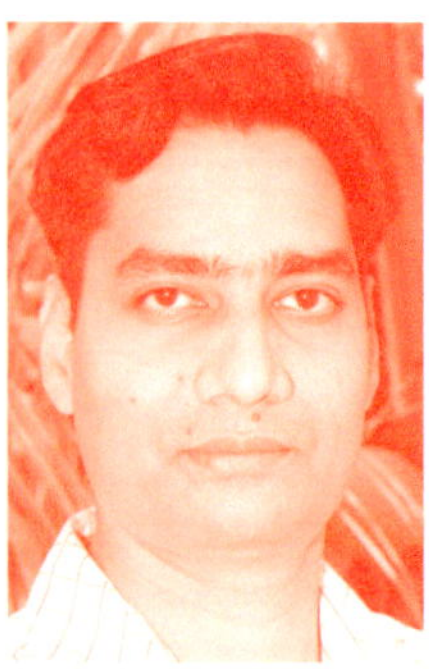
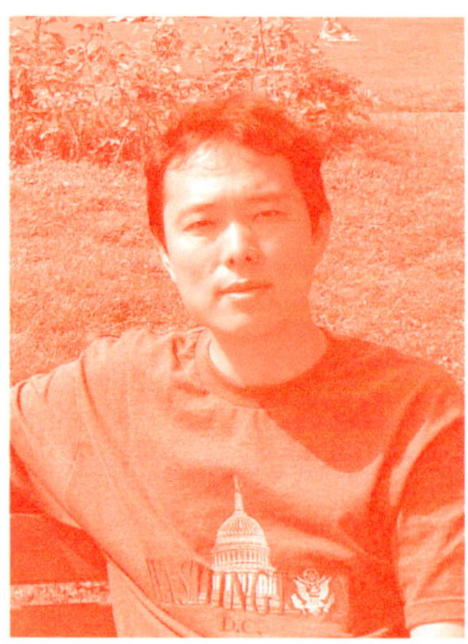
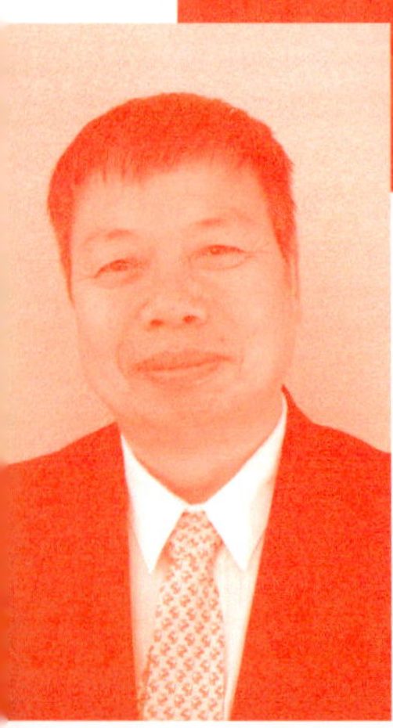
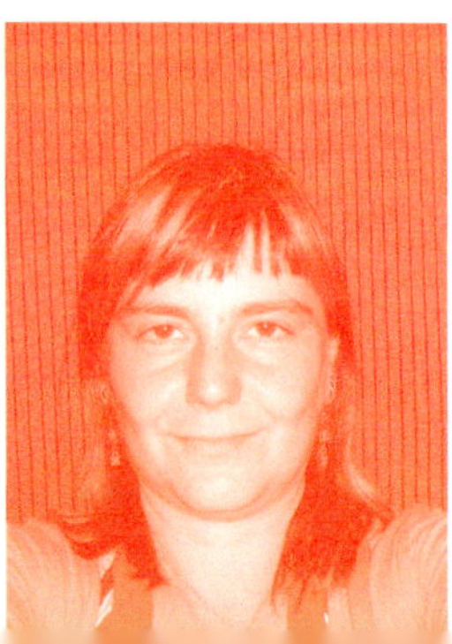

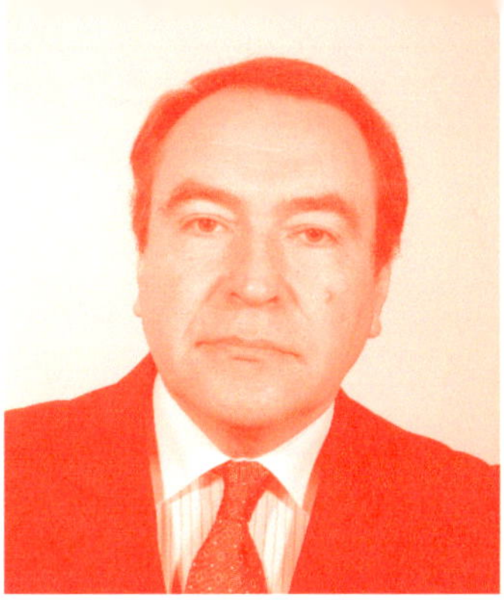
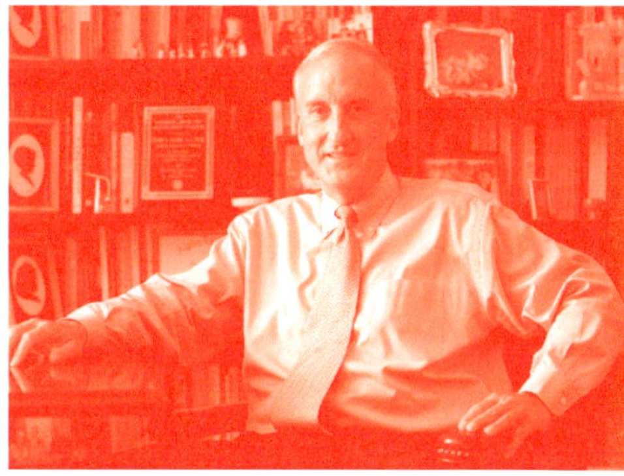
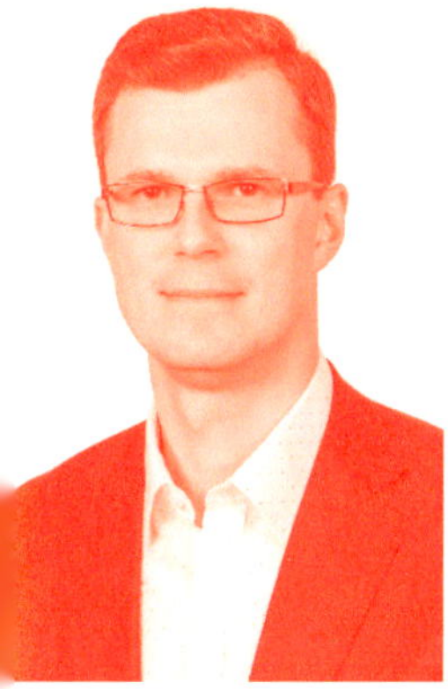
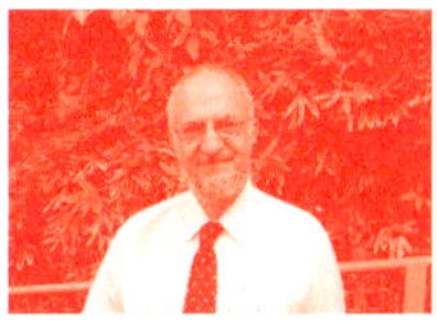
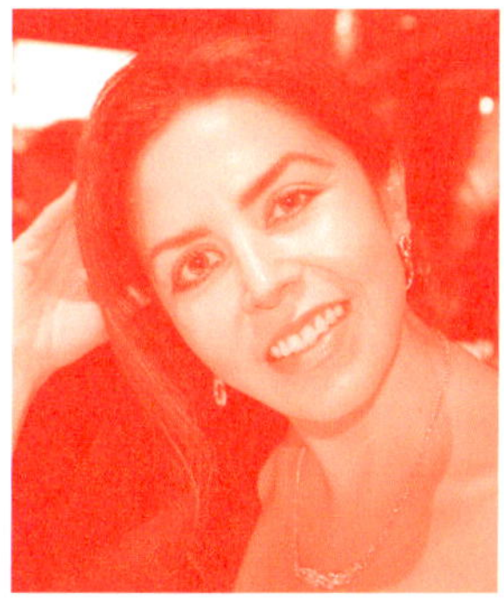

Supporting open minds since 2005

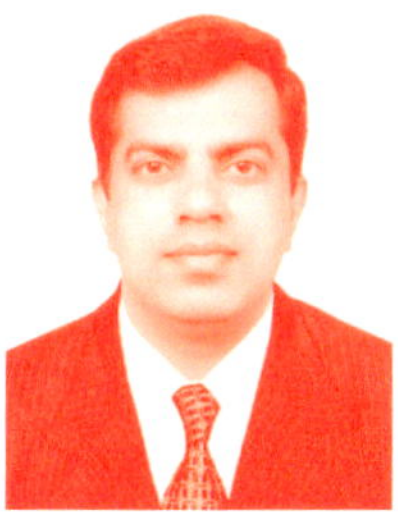
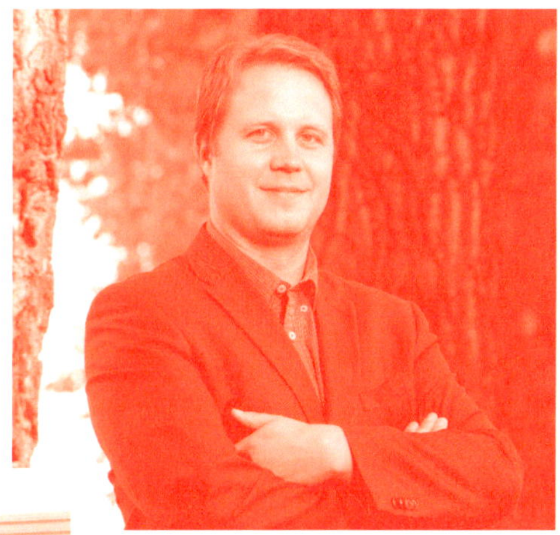
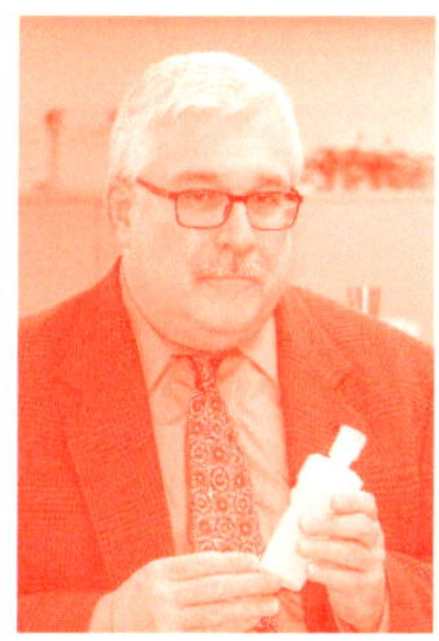
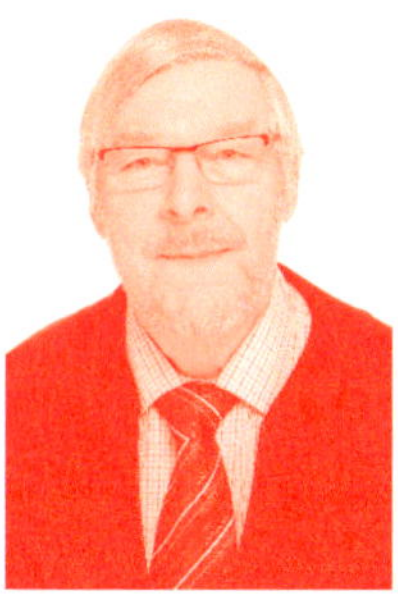
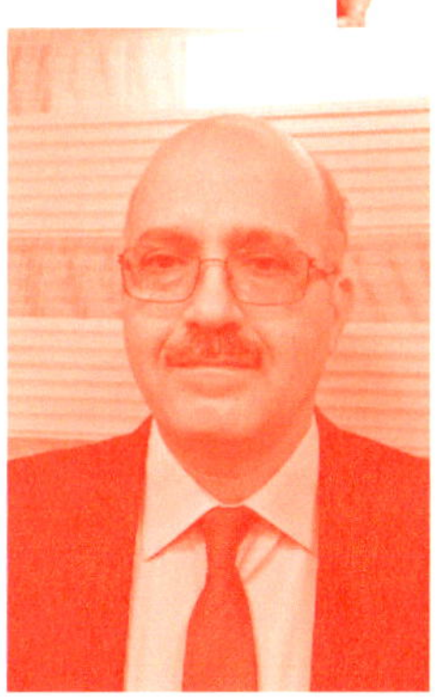
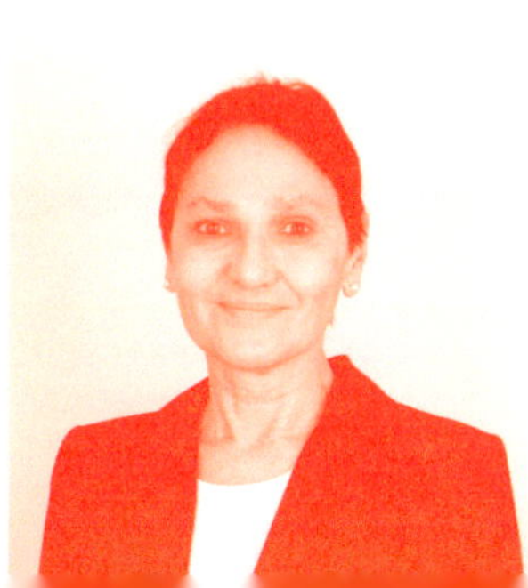
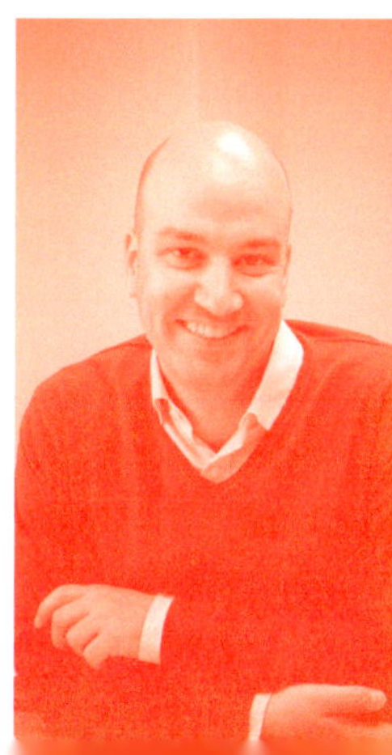

Wound Healing
http://dx.doi.org/10.5772/intechopen.83061
Edited by Muhammad Ahmad

Contributors
Juin-Hong Cherng, Lydmila Antipova, Sergey Titov, Stanislav Storublevtcev, Sergey Antipov, V. V. Loboda, M.S. Bolokov, M.G. Khatkhokhu, Ji-Cheng Hsieh, Robert Galiano, Chitang Joshi, Abbas Hassan, Jesus Escriva-Machado, Eduardo Camacho-Quintero, Alejandro Maciel-Miranda, Julia De La Luz-Hernanadez, Samuel Almeida-Navarro, Felipe De Sousa, Francisco Rogênio Da Silva Mendes, Jose Jovanny Bermudez-Sierra, Ayrles Fernanda Brandão Da Silva, Mirele Da Silveira Vasconcelos, Tamiris De Fátima Goebel De Souza, Marília De Oliveira Nunes, Antônio Eufrásio Vieira-Neto, Marcos Roberto Lourenzoni, Rosueti Diógenes De Oliveira-Filho, Adriana Rolim Campos, Renato De Azevedo Moreira, Ana Cristina De Oliveira Monteiro-Moreira, Diptiman Choudhury, Pawandeep Kaur, Maria Marques, Eglantina Afonso, Dina Borges, Kátia Furtado, Margarida Pedro, Inês Reis, Rita Morais

First published in London, United Kingdom, 2020 by IntechOpen
IntechOpen is the global imprint of INTECHOPEN LIMITED, registered in England and Wales, registration number: 11086078, 7th floor, 10 Lower Thames Street, London, EC3R 6AF, United Kingdom
Printed in Croatia

British Library Cataloguing-in-Publication Data
A catalogue record for this book is available from the British Library

Additional hard and PDF copies can be obtained from orders@intechopen.com

Wound Healing
Edited by Muhammad Ahmad
p. cm.
Print ISBN 978-1-78985-957-7
Online ISBN 978-1-78985-958-4
eBook (PDF) ISBN 978-1-83880-965-2

For EU product safety concerns:
IN TECH d.o.o., Prolaz Marije Krucifikse Kozulić 3, 51000 Rijeka, Croatia, info@intechopen.com or visit our website at intechopen.com.

Meet the editor

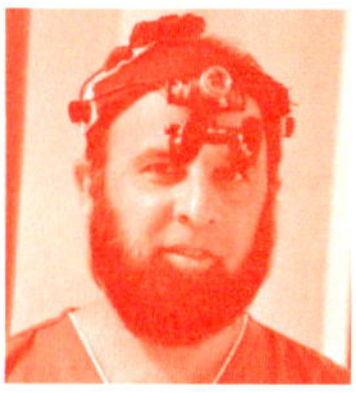

Dr. Muhammad Ahmad is the only surgeon in history to develop various new classifications regarding different aspects of hair restoration. These include a new classification system for hair loss, Ahmad's NPRT system; a new classification for scalp hair, LGMA classification; and a comprehensive classification of hair transection. He has also published Ahmad's Cosmetic Surgery Scar Scale and Ahmad's Hair Transplant Assessment Scale. He is the only Pakistani plastic surgeon to receive the Merit Award from the Australian and New Zealand Burns Association (2004). He was also awarded first prize at the annual meeting of the Asian Association of Hair Restoration Surgeons (AAHRS), Bangkok, Thailand, in 2017. In 2018, he was awarded a Lifetime Achievement Award from the Pakistan Society of Hair Restoration Surgery. Dr. Ahmad has more than 125 publications in national and international journals. He is also editor and reviewer of many international journals.

Contents

Preface

I am honored to serve as editor of *Wound Healing* from IntechOpen publishing. Wound healing is a vast subject and this book presents recent information and basic knowledge about wound management, including healing mechanisms and actions.

Chapters cover such topics as negative pressure wound management, hypertrophic scarring, biomaterials derived from plants, insulin use, and modified collagen.

This book will help dermatologists, students, surgeons, and physicians who treat patients with wounds. It provides a comprehensive overview of the subject, including pathophysiology and clinical and medical management.

I would like to thank my wife Nabila and my two sons, Muhammad and Muhammad Abdullah, who supported me during the various stages of preparing this manuscript.

Dr. Muhammad Ahmad, MD
Plastic and Hair Restoration Surgeon,
Aesthetic Plastic Surgery and Hair Transplant Institute,
Islamabad, Pakistan

Section 1

Basic Sciences and Clinical Approaches

Chapter 1

Calcium Alginate Polysaccharide Dressing as an Accelerated Treatment for Burn Wound Healing

Juin-Hong Cherng

Abstract

Patients with burn injuries suffer from pain and an inflammatory response; however, treatment methods are still not satisfactory and remain challenging. Due to the long stage of burn wound rehabilitation, which contributes to the long-term sensory problems, an effective treatment must begin at the outset of burn wound care. The functionalized wound dressing is expected to be a great treatment strategy over the commercialization wound dressing products and engineered skin substitutes nowadays. Some studies revealed the use of calcium alginate polysaccharide (CAPS) as an "active" dressing due to its calcium richness for wound healing and scar tissue formation. The outstanding outcome of CAPS dressing for severe burn injuries was indicated by natural wound healing and less scarring formation, minimum bacterial infection, cytokine enhancement regulation, and appropriate inflammatory response and pain regulation. These advantages affirmed the phyto-polysaccharide dressing as the next generation of wound dressing materials with highly desirable properties.

Keywords: severe burn injuries, wound dressing, wound management, calcium alginate polysaccharide, inflammatory response

1. Introduction

Burns are the most traumatic injuries and physically harmful because of long hospitalization and rehabilitation, which lead to significant morbidity and mortality [1, 2]. The development of effective treatment associated with burn injury is a major unmet medical problem. Current burn wound treatment methods, such as eschar excision, split-thickness skin autograft, and cell-based skin constructs, are still not satisfactory and remain challenging. Not only causing painful and relative costly treatment, but those methods are also very difficult to perform in patients due to poor availability of healthy tissue [3–5].

Despite any advances in burn management, how to treat wound properly at the outset of burn injury is the important key of an effective treatment. Most patients with burn injuries suffer from long-term pain and posttraumatic situation; therefore, an appropriate burn wound handling with a good dressing initially is expected to be a great way to minimize scar formation and accelerate burn wound healing.

IntechOpen

A good clinical dressing must be easy to handle, avoids infection and inflammation, has no toxicity, causes no allergic reactions, and permits easy and early mobilization [6, 7].

Bioactive wound dressing, or functionalized wound dressing, is expected to overcome the limitations of the current treatment in burn wound management. This dressing delivers either bioactive compounds or dressing that is constructed from a material having endogenous activity in wound healing, which contribute not only a matrix for repair but also growth factors and cytokines to enhance the healing process [8]. Various types of bioactive wound dressings are available on the market and are used clinically. However, bioactive wound dressings have advantages and disadvantages, so choosing the suitable wound dressing as needed is advised.

Alginate, commonly derived from seaweed, has been widely investigated by many researchers for possible new alternative in wound management field. Alginate, a rich natural polysaccharide, which contains glycosaminoglycan (GAG), has several major properties such as biocompatibility, gelling, and swelling that keep the wound site moist enough for proper healing and then able to reduce healing times of wounds [9, 10]. When attached with wound, an ion-exchange reaction occurs between the calcium in the alginate and the sodium in the exudate, thus producing a soluble gel that help maintain a moist wound environment and also hold bacterial infection in absorbed wound fluid at the same time. This is why alginate is recommended for the treatment of moderate to highly exuding wounds [11].

Calcium alginate polysaccharide (CAPS) has been found suitable for use in pharmaceutical drugs, as a bioactive food ingredient, and for cell encapsulation or tissue regeneration [12]. Numerous studies revealed that CAPS-containing dressing for severe burn injuries has outstanding outcomes such as rapid wound closure with less scarring formation, minimum bacterial infection, cytokine enhancement regulation, and appropriate inflammatory response and pain regulation. In addition, this material becomes substantial to be considered as optimal burn wound dressing treatment because it maintains a great moist microenvironment at the wound site. Therefore, the detail mechanisms and involvement of CAPS dressing in accelerating burn wound healing will be further discussed in this chapter.

2. Medical dressing for the treatment of burn injury

Generally, the treatment of burn injury depends on both depth and surface area of burn wounds, which reepithelialization is the most important stage of burn wound repair. For the severe burn injury such as deep partial-thickness or full-thickness burn, there is a need of special treatment to prevent delayed reepithelialization due to the destruction of epithelial regenerative elements in the basal layer of the epidermis and in the dermis. To date, eschar excision and split-thickness skin autograft taken from a healthy skin of the same patient are medical standard treatments for severe burn injury [3, 4]. However, the grafts are causing pain and very difficult to perform in patients due to poor availability of healthy tissue. In addition, many types of cell-based skin constructs have been developed for full-thickness burn injury, but poor survival rate of the keratinocytes in cell sheets has been a major concern in these discoveries [5].

On the other hand, for the first or superficial second-degree injury, the reepithelialization remains possible by the migration of keratinocytes from the edges of the wound, followed by their proliferation, stratification, and dedifferentiation to form an intact epithelium [3]. But still, an optimal reepithelialization requires a supportive microenvironment to avoid infection. Bacterial infection was well known as a common cause of death after burns [13]. Commonly, antimicrobial creams and occlusive dressings are applied on the wound to avoid infection, to limit wound progression, and to improve epithelialization progression [14].

Despite any advances in burn management, how to treat wound properly at the outset of burn injury is the important key of an effective treatment. The proper burn wound handling in the beginning with the functionalized wound dressing may enhance reepithelialization progress and accelerate an intact epithelium formation with minimal scar appearance. Not only should achieve rapid healing at reasonable cost with less inconvenience to the patient, but the use of clinical dressing also must be easy to handle, avoids infection and inflammation, has no toxicity, causes no allergic reactions, and permits easy and early mobilization [6, 7].

Based on its natural action, wound dressings are normally classified as passive products, interactive products, and bioactive products [9]. Passive products consist of traditional dressings like gauze and tulle dressings which account for the largest market segment. Interactive products consist of polymeric films and forms, which are recommended for low exuding wounds due to its characteristics. Bioactive products are which deliver either bioactive compounds or dressings are constructed from a material having endogenous activity in wound healing. These materials include proteoglycans, collagen, non-collagenous protein, chitosan, or alginate. They are considered to contribute not only a matrix for repair but also growth factors and cytokines to enhance the healing process [8]. Commercially, various types of those bioactive wound dressings are currently used in the clinical setting with their advantages and disadvantages for some types of wounds. In the case of burn wound, the dressing with rich glycosaminoglycan (GAG) is expected to encourage the efficient and rapid healing process. GAG has a significant role in wound healing phases which acts as a regulator of early inflammation to modulate inflammatory cell and fibroblast cell migration, pro-inflammatory cytokine synthesis, and the phagocytosis of invading microbes [15].

Alginate, commonly derived from seaweed, is a rich natural anionic phytol polysaccharide (APS) that consists of mainly differing ratios of D-mannuronic and L-guluronic acid, which are covalently bound through 1,4-glycosidic linkages. Polysaccharides and proteins are the most common natural polymers used in the tissue engineering field for the regeneration of full-thickness wounds because of their biocompatibility, biodegradability, and similarity with ECM [16, 17]. Containing glycosaminoglycan (GAG), they play a key role in wound healing due to their ability to encourage activation of the immune system that cleans up the wound site after injury and reduces the pain simultaneously. It provides a moist environment around the wound site that leads to rapid granulation and reepithelialization. Alginate-based wound dressings have also been demonstrated for their hemostatic properties in exudation/bleeding wounds and burns [9]. Alginate can easily form gels by binding with divalent cations, especially calcium ions [18]. The gelling property of alginate helps in the dressing removal without much trauma [19].

Alginate dressings were originally presented as formed from calcium alginate fibers and have been technically fabricated with fibers woven to form a more solid and strengthen structure to obtain an applicable wound dressing. As wound dressing, treatment with calcium alginate polysaccharide (CAPS) dressings had shown great wound recovery outcome in various types of skin wounds [20–23]. They promoted healing via a direct modulatory effect on wound macrophage activation that secretes pro-inflammatory cytokines within the chronic wound bed which may initiate a delayed inflammatory phase [24]. Additionally, numerous studies revealed that CAPS-containing dressing for severe burn injuries has outstanding outcomes such as rapid wound closure with less scarring formation, minimum bacterial infection, cytokine enhancement regulation, and appropriate inflammatory response and pain regulation. Hence, this material becomes substantial to be considered as an optimal burn wound dressing.

3. The problem and historical perspective of burn wound healing

The proper treatment of wound has attracted the human attention over several decades. Among the various types of wound, severe burn injuries are the most traumatic and physically harmful, which lead to significant morbidity and mortality [1, 2]. Burn injuries can lead to multifarious uncontrolled effects after the accident, and they may have a major impact to the body functions of burn-injured patients. Historically, they were accounted for an estimate of 180,000 deaths every year, which are related to burn injury worldwide, and the vast majority occurs in low- and middle-income countries [25]. Most burn victims face up a long-term hospitalization and suffer major burns covering 25% of their body surface.

The healing process of burn wound, both small burn and large severe burn injuries, occurs through several biological processes, such as hemostasis, inflammation, proliferation, and maturation. Without the right handling, a hypertrophic scar caused by fibroblastic proliferation will be formed during the healing process, which is confined to the wound site [26]. In addition to local wound repair, severe large burns also can stimulate a persistent pathophysiological stress response [27]. Most patients with burn injuries suffer pain during burn wound debridement in the clinic, which they describe as severe to excruciating despite the use of powerful opioid analgesics [28]. Based on local and systemic pathophysiologic responses, burn wound recovery is generally divided into three phases: acute phase, healing phase, and rehabilitation phase. The acute phase may be completely bypassed in smaller injuries, which specifically lasts 2–3 days [29, 30]; the healing phase may be weeks or more, whereas the rehabilitation phase most often takes at least 1 year and sometimes much longer, depending on patient participation in the treatment plan, patient age, and specification of burn [31]. These long phases of recovery often lead burn-injured patients to survive from long-term pain and encounter a posttraumatic situation.

In order to reduce the lifelong burn wound recovery phases which usually contributes to the further problems, an effective treatment must begin at the outset of burn wound care. An appropriate burn wound handling in the beginning is expected to be a great way to minimize scar formation and accelerate burn wound healing.

4. Application of CAPS dressing for accelerating burn injury treatment

Since burns have a heterogeneous nature, a variety of animal burn models have been developed as valuable tools to observe the pathophysiology of burns. Animal models continue to be explored to uncover the molecular and cellular aspects that characterize human burn trauma [32]. Better understanding of the burn wound healing in animal models and their relation to human wounds will significantly overcome the limited translation of research into practical treatments for burn-injured patients.

Wang et al. [33] treated a severe burn injury in swine model with calcium alginate polysaccharide (CAPS) dressing to observe wound repair and scar formation comparing to the use of carboxymethyl cellulose (CMC) as a commonly used wound dressing for many years [34, 35]. These animals were also used to assess the secondary outcomes of the depth of scar formation at postburn, determined by the Vancouver Scar Scale (VSS) which consists of four variables: vascularity, height (thickness), pliability, and pigmentation. The total score ranges from 0 to 14, whereby a score of 0 reflects normal skin. The results showed that wounds dressed with CAPS exhibit a rapid reepithelialization and less scar formation, which appeared with a smooth wound. Based on VSS scores, there was less scar formation in the wounds dressed with CAPS, shown by significantly lower scores up to 6 weeks of observation. Scarring, or fibrosis, is known as an abnormal tissue remodeling. The management of scar formation is one of major complications encountered during the wound healing process. Without the right handling, a hypertrophic scar caused by fibroblastic proliferation will be formed during the healing process [26]. Moreover, healing by fibrosis instead of regeneration often causes lifelong disability that has a significant economic impact [36].

In line, an obvious wound closure and relative complete reepithelialization were observed to occur on wound dressed with the CAPS dressing in rat group model [37]. Their histological analysis revealed that the new dermis tissue on dressing treated wound area was composed of reorganized and stratified epithelial layer, with fully developed connective tissue, hair follicle, sebaceous glands, and aligned collagen. Another study reported that CAPS dressing treatment accelerated wound closure rate and exhibited a faster epithelialization [38]. They found that the expression of skin tissue collagen I was elevated by CAPS dressing application, and this dressing provides a moist environment and a faster collagen I-related epithelialization.

The ability of CAPS dressing reduces scar formation in burn injury is attributable to its rich contain of glycosaminoglycan (GAG), which was known to promote wound healing, lead to rapid granulation and reepithelialization, and thus yield a minimum scar formation certainly. Moreover, when attached to the wound, an ion-exchange reaction occurs between the calcium in the alginate and the sodium in the exudate, producing a soluble gel that turns to help maintain a moist wound environment [39]. CAPS dressings also have their inherent ability to augment hemostasis, as release of calcium ions leads to platelet activation [40, 41]. Additionally, calcium ions also speed up the wound healing process by modulating cell proliferation, maturation, and the creation of epidermal lipid barriers [42–44].

As another major challenge in burn injury management, bacterial infection becomes the most common cause of mortality and morbidity [13, 45, 46]. Infection is defined as the presence of high concentrations ($>10^5$ organisms/g of tissue) of bacteria in the burn wound and usually progresses to invasion of subjacent tissue within 5 days. Infection can delay wound healing process due to the development of a pronounced immune response, accompanied by sepsis or septic shock, which causes hypotension and impaired perfusion of end organs including the skin. To prevent this condition, wound dressing for burn injury treatment should create an optimal environment, which provides barrier against chronic wound infection.

Some studies have demonstrated that CAPS dressings have hemostatic [47] and some bacteriostatic [48] properties. CAPS dressing for burn wound treatment demonstrated a remarkable inhibition of bacterial growth than CMC dressing treatment, which significantly reduced the amount of bacteria at 3 weeks postburn injury [33]. This reduction was maintained until 6 weeks postburn injury. The infection control functioned by CAPS dressing might be related to its bacterial infection holding in absorbed wound fluid. As they swell, they trap wound debris and bacteria, thereby reducing overall bacterial load within the wound during dressing changes [19]. In addition, the advantages of a new technology conferring a bactericidal effect on CAPS gels for wound dressing have been explored. Poor et al. [49] developed nonthermal-plasma-treated alginate gel wound dressing, and the results showed that this treatment has better wound decontamination and wound healing capabilities, as well as broad-spectrum antibacterial activity and negligible cytotoxicity.

CAPS dressing reduced the bacterial growth through the release of calcium, which has been recommended as an antimicrobial agent [50–55], resulting in superior bactericidal and bacteriolytic effects compared with other antimicrobial agents [52–55]. Moreover, the use of alginate derivatives such as antibacterial, antiviral, and antifungal agents has been revealed by numerous data [56, 57]. Negatively charged alginates were found to interact with the outer bacterial cellular surface, which causes disruption and leakage of intracellular substances [58, 59]. Additionally, the ability of alginate modulating the production of toxins, microbial growth, and factors crucial for microorganism's stability could be the reasons for its antibacterial efficacy characteristic. Some varieties of bacteria such as *Pseudomonas*, *Escherichia*, *Proteus*, and *Acinetobacter* have been proven to be detained by bacteriostatic activity of alginate [60, 61].

Further, the CAPS dressing treatment has also demonstrated its critical role in inflammation. Inflammation is a crucial stage to successful burn wound healing. The release of pro-inflammatory cytokines, such as interleukin (IL)-1β, IL-6, IL-8, interferon (INF)-γ, and tumor necrosis factor (TNF)-α, after thermal injury is one of the important systemic inflammatory responses in burn-induced skin damages [62, 63]. Pro-/anti-inflammatory cytokines act as important modulators of immune cell proliferation, differentiation, and clonal growth of lymphocyte subpopulations and also attract immune cells to the site of burn injuries [64], which are substantial in the process of burn wound recovery.

The involvement of IL-4, IL-6, TNF-α, and MCP-1 was found in the early stages of the rat's response to burn injury treated with CAPS dressing [33]. Immune cells were attracted by these cytokines to the site of injuries to initiate an immune response right away after burning. The ratio of IL-6 to TNF-α can be used to predict mortality from sepsis following burn injury [65]. IL-4 and IL-8 may serve as predictive biomarkers of mortality from sepsis and/or multiple organ failure (MOF) [66]. In addition, MCP-1, an initiator of typ. 2 T-cell generation and an indicator of bacterial infection, is essential for optimal microbial elimination [52]. The involvement of MCP-1 in Gram-positive bacterial infections has been demonstrated in the control of *Listeria monocytogenes* infections [53]. Chan et al. [67] and Thomas et al. [24] have also revealed the similar results both in vitro and in vivo. Particularly, aside from the other chemokines and cytokines, at least fivefold more of IL-1β secretion was found from CAPS gel treatment compared to agarose and collagen gel treatment [67]. IL-1β is known as a critical mediator of inflammation which has substantial roles in neutrophil mobilization, cellular adhesion to the endothelium, and white blood cell infiltration [68, 69].

Furthermore, the pain is related with the modulation of transforming growth factor (TGF-β), an important inflammatory cytokine and anti-inflammatory factor [70–72], that implicated in the pathogenesis of keloids and hypertrophic scarring. TGF-β also participates in the mechanism of pain signals including peripheral and central processing [71]. CAPS dressing for burn wound treatment demonstrated high levels of TGF-β1, TGF-β2, and TGF-β3, suggesting that it might contribute to reduced pain perception [33]. TGF-β1 is responsible for the fibrotic scarring response, whereas TGF-β2 and TGF-β3 are responsible for the scarless wound healing [70]. Another study confirmed that alginate-containing dressings can augment natural wound healing with inhibition of cytokines associated with fibrosis, resulting in decreased wound size and increasing epithelial proliferation [73].

Those data correlated very well with the use of CAPS dressing for human skin wound in the clinical setting recently. CAPS dressings were applied after perianal abscess surgery, which was known as an acute suppurative infectious disease that occurs around the anus, anal canal, and rectum. The results showed that the expression of a variety of proliferative cytokines increases in the wound treated with CAPS dressing and helps promote wound healing [74]. The CAPS dressing treatment also was found to increase the synthesis of collagen and, on the other hand, inhibit the apoptosis of mitochondrial pathway and death receptor pathway.

Some literatures revealed that calcium ions from Ca-alginate systems [62] and oligosaccharides derived from polysaccharides (β-glucan, xyloglucan, chitin, pectin, D-mannuronic, and L-guluronic) can stimulate human cells to produce cytokines [75, 76]. Especially, enhancement of IL-1β secretion was expected due to the connection between calcium ion-induced mitochondrial damage and activation of the NLRP3 inflammasome, an important molecular platform expressed by myeloid cells in innate immune defense [77–79]. Besides, alginate-containing dressings have the potential to activate macrophages and have the ability to generate a pro-inflammatory signal which promotes granulation tissue formation [24]. However, another factor that may be important in cytokine induction not only relates to the proportions of guluronic to mannuronic acid residues but also their polymeric arrangement [80].

In summary, because of these properties, CAPS dressings are considered as a bioactive wound dressing and expected to accelerate the treatment for burn wound healing. There were few products made from CAPS related to surgery and wound management previously but, due to the small amount of these fibers used in total product with high-cost manufacture, it seems not profitable to continue the production. With the improved technology lately, CAPS has been developed into spinning fine dressing as an applicable wound dressing. Together with the increased understanding of CAPS beneficials in accelerating burn injury treatment, it is expected that CAPS dressing will give potential value for medical and business field simultaneously.

5. Conclusion

As the glycosaminoglycan (GAG) has influential roles in the stimulation of rapid wound healing, calcium alginate polysaccharide (CAPS), which contains a rich amount of GAG, can be regarded as a remarkable material-based wound dressing option. Since this material had technically actualized into spinning fibers woven or non-woven, it is expected that CAPS-containing wound dressing not only gives an optimal burn injury treatment alternative in medical field but also can rise up the textile industry value from the business perspective. Owing the significant benefits as an “active” dressing for burn wound recovery, such as rapid wound closure with less scarring formation, minimum bacterial infection, cytokine enhancement regulation, and appropriate inflammatory response and pain regulation, which have been demonstrated in several studies and clinical trials, therefore, the CAPS dressing holds a promising potential as the advisable preference of burn injury treatment strategies with highly desirable properties.

Acknowledgements

The author would like to thank Dr. Chih-Hsin Wang (Department of Plastic and Reconstructive Surgery) and Dr. Cheng-Che Liu (Department of Physiology and Biophysics, Graduate Institute of Physiology) at Tri-Service General Hospital,

National Defense Medical Center, Taipei, Taiwan (ROC), for their helpful discussion during this chapter writing.

Conflict of interest

The author declared no potential conflicts of interest with respect to the research, authorship, and/or publication of this article.

Author details

Juin-Hong Cherng[1,2,3]*

1 Department and Graduate Institute of Biology and Anatomy, National Defense Medical Center, Taipei, Taiwan, ROC

2 General Clinical Research Center for New Drug Trial, Tri-Service General Hospital, National Defense Medical Center, Taipei, Taiwan, ROC

3 Department of Gerontological Health Care, National Taipei University of Nursing and Health Sciences, Taipei, Taiwan, ROC

*Address all correspondence to: i72bbb@gmail.com

References

[1] Sanchez JL, Pereperez SB, Bastida JL, Martinez MM. Cost-utility analysis applied to the treatment of burn patients in a specialized center. Archives of Surgery. 2007;**142**:50-57. DOI: 10.1001/archsurg.142.1.50

[2] de Roche R, Luscher NJ, Debrunner HU, Fischer R. Epidemiological data and costs of burn injuries in workers in Switzerland: An argument for immediate treatment in burn centers. Burns. 1994;**20**:58-60. DOI: 10.1016/0305-4179(94)90108-2

[3] Papini R. Management of burn injuries of various depths. BMJ. 2004; **329**:158. DOI: 10.1136/bmj.329.7458.158

[4] Andreassi A, Bilenchi R, Biagioli M, D'Aniello C. Classification and pathophysiology of skin grafts. Clinics in Dermatology. 2005;**23**:332. DOI: 10.1016/j.clindermatol.2004.07.024

[5] Odessey R. Addendum: Multicenter experience with cultured epidermal autograft for treatment of burns. The Journal of Burn Care & Rehabilitation. 1992;**13**(1):174-180. DOI: 10.1097/00004630-199201000-00038

[6] Reig A, Tejerina C, Codina J, Hidalgo J, Mirabet V. Application of a new cicatrization dressing in treating second-degree burns and donor sites. Annals of the MBC. 1991;**4**:174-176

[7] Hindy A. Comparative study between sodium carboxymethyl-cellulose silver, moist exposed burn ointment, and saline-soaked dressing for treatment of facial burns. Annals of Burns and Fire Disasters. 2009;**22**: 131-137. PMID: 21991168

[8] Stashak TS, Farstvedt E, Othic A. Update on wound dressings: Indications and best use. Clinical Techniques in Equine Practice. 2004;**3**(2):148-163. DOI: 10.1053/j.ctep.2004.08.006

[9] Sweeney IR, Miraftab M, Collyer G. A critical review of modern and emerging absorbent dressings used to treat exuding wounds. International Wound Journal. 2012;**9**(6):601-612. DOI: 10.1111/j.1742-481X.2011.00923.x

[10] Fan L, Li M, Gong Y, Peng K, Xie W. Preparation and characterization of alginate/Hydroxypropyl chitosan blend fibers. Journal of Applied Polymer Science. 2012;**125**(2):829-835. DOI: 10.1002/app.35629

[11] Andersen T, Markussen C, Dornish M, et al. In situ gelation for cell immobilization and culture in alginate foam scaffolds. Tissue Engineering. Part A. 2014;**20**(3–4):600-610. DOI: 10.1089/ten.TEA.2013.0223

[12] Matricardi P, Meo CD, Coviello T, Alhaique F. Recent advances and perspectives on coated alginate microspheres for modified drug delivery. Expert Opinion on Drug Delivery. 2008;**5**:417-425. DOI: 10.1517/17425247.5.4.417

[13] D'Avignon LC, Hogan BK, Murray CK, Loo FL, Hospenthal DR, et al. Contribution of bacterial and viral infections to attributable mortality in patients with severe burns: An autopsy series. Burns. 2010;**36**:773-779. DOI: 10.1016/j.burns.2009.11.007

[14] Sevgi M, Toklu A, Vecchio D, Hamblin MR. Topical antimicrobials for burn infections-an update. Recent Patents on Anti-Infective Drug Discovery. 2013;**8**(3):161-197. DOI: 10.2174/1574891X08666131112143447

[15] Chen WY, Abatangelo G. Functions of hyaluronan in wound repair. Wound Repair and Regeneration. 1999;7(2):

79-89. DOI: 10.1046/j.1524-475X.1999.00079.x

[16] Malafaya PB, Silva GA, Reis RL. Natural-origin polymers as carriers and scaffolds for biomolecules and cell delivery in tissue engineering applications. Advanced Drug Delivery Reviews. 2007;**59**:207-233. DOI: 10.1016/j.addr.2007.03.012

[17] Wiegand C, Hipler UC. Polymer-based biomaterials as dressings for chronic stagnating wounds. Macromolecular Symposia. 2010;**294**: 1-13. DOI: 10.1002/masy.200900028

[18] LeRoux MA, Guilak F, Setton LA. Compressive and shear properties of alginate gel: Effects of sodium ions and alginate concentration. Journal of Biomedical Materials Research. 1999; **47**(1):46-53. DOI: 10.1002/(SICI)1097-4636(199910)47:13.0.CO;2-N

[19] Fanucci D, Seese J. Multi-faceted use of calcium alginates. A painless, cost-effective alternative for wound care management. OWM. 1991;**37**:16-22. PMID: 1764155

[20] Bale S, Baker N, Crook H, Rayman A, Rayman G, Harding KG. Exploring the use of an alginate dressing for diabetic foot ulcers. Journal of Wound Care. 2001;**10**(3):81-84. DOI: 10.12968/jowc.2001.10.3.26063

[21] Sayag J, Meaume S, Bohbot S. Healing properties of calcium alginate dressings. Journal of Wound Care. 1996; **5**(8):357-362. DOI: 10.12968/jowc.1996.5.8.357

[22] Attwood AI. Calcium alginate dressing accelerates split skin graft donor site healing. British Journal of Plastic Surgery. 1989;**42**(4):373-379. DOI: 10.1016/0007-1226(89)90001-5

[23] Kneafsey B, O'Shaughnessy M, Condon KC. The use of calcium alginate dressings in deep hand burns. Burns. 1996;**22**(1):40-43. DOI: 10.1016/0305-4179(95)00066-6

[24] Thomas A, Harding KG, Moore K. Alginates from wound dressings activate human macrophages to secrete tumour necrosis factor-alpha. Biomaterials. 2000;**21**:797-802. DOI: 10.1016/S0142-9612(00)00072-7

[25] WHO. Burns: 2018 update [Internet]. 2018. Available from: http://www.who.int/mediacentre/factsheets/fs365/en/ [Accessed: 10 April 2018]

[26] Eming SA, Martin P, Tomic-Canic M. Wound repair and regeneration: Mechanisms, signaling, and translation. Science Translational Medicine. 2014;**6**: 265-266. DOI: 10.1126/scitranslmed.3009337

[27] Wang Y, Beekman J, Hew J, Jackson S, Issler-Fisher AC, Parungao R, et al. Burn injury: Challenges and advances in burn wound healing, infection, pain and scarring. Advanced Drug Delivery Reviews. 2018;**123**:3-17. DOI: 10.1016/j.addr.2017.09.018

[28] Verhaegen PD, van Zuijlen PP, Pennings NM, van Marle J, Niessen FB, van der Horst CM, et al. Differences in collagen architecture between keloid, hypertrophic scar, normotrophic scar, and normal skin: An objective histopathological analysis. Wound Repair and Regeneration. 2009;**17**: 649-656. DOI: 10.1111/j.1524-475X.2009.00533.x

[29] Meyer WJ, Marvin JA, Patterson DR, Thomas C, Blakeney PE. Management of pain and other discomforts in burned patients. In: Herndon D, editor. Handbook of Total Burn Care. 2nd ed. London: WB Saunders; 2001. pp. 747-765

[30] Ready LB, Edwards WT. Handbook of Management of Acute Pain: A Practical Guide. Seattle, WA:

International Association for the Study of Pain (IASP); 1992

[31] Lauterbach S, George R. Burn pain. In: McCaffrey M, Pasero C, editors. Handbook of Pain: Clinical Manual. St. Louis, MO: Mosby; 1999. pp. 527-531

[32] Jakubowski K, Poellmann M, Lee RC. Precision burn trauma medicine: Application for molecular engineering science. Engineering. 2015;1(3):280–281. DOI: 10.15302/J-ENG-2015073

[33] Wang CH, Chang SJ, Tzeng YS, Shih YJ, Adrienne C, Chen SG, et al. Enhanced wound-healing performance of a phyto-polysaccharide-enriched dressing-a preclinical small and large animal study. International Wound Journal. 2017;**14**:1359-1369. DOI: 10.1111/iwj.12813

[34] Biswal DR, Singh RP. Characterisation of carboxymethyl cellulose and polyacrylamide graft copolymer. Carbohydrate Polymers. 2004;**57**:379-387. DOI: 10.1016/j.carbpol.2004.04.020

[35] Fan L, Zhou X, Wu P, Xie W, Zheng H, Tan W, et al. Preparation of carboxymethyl cellulose sulfates and its application as anticoagulant and wound dressing. International Journal of Biological Macromolecules. 2014;**66**:245-253. DOI: 10.1016/j.ijbiomac.2014.02.040

[36] Aarabi S, Longaker MT, Gurtner GC. Hypertrophic scar formation following burns and trauma: New approaches to treatment. PLoS Medicine. 2007;**4**(9):e234. DOI: 10.1371/journal.pmed.0040234

[37] Liu X, Liu H, Qu X, Lei M, Zhang C, Hong H, et al. Electrical signals triggered controllable formation of calcium alginate film for wound treatment. Journal of Materials Science: Materials in Medicine. 2017;**28**:146. DOI: 10.1007/s10856-017-5956-x

[38] Wang T, Gu Q, Zhao J, Mei J, Shao M, Pan Y, et al. Calcium alginate enhances wound healing by up-regulating the ratio of collagen types I/III in diabetic rats. International Journal of Clinical and Experimental Pathology. 2015;**8**(6):6636-6645. PMID: 26261545

[39] Kannon GA, Garrett AB. Moist wound healing with occlusive dressings. A clinical review. Dermatologic Surgery. 1995;**21**:583-590. DOI: 10.1111/j.1524-4725.1995.tb00511.x

[40] Segal HC, Hunt BJ, Gilding K. The effects of alginate and non-alginate wound dressings on blood coagulation and platelet activation. Journal of Biomaterials Applications. 1998;**12**:249-257. DOI: 10.1177/088532829801200305

[41] Barnett SE, Varley SJ. The effects of calcium alginate on wound healing. Annals of the Royal College of Surgeons of England. 1987;**69**:153-155. PMID: 3631870

[42] Sun L, Huang Y, Bian Z, Petrosino J, Fan Z, Wang Y, et al. Sundew-inspired adhesive hydrogels combined with adipose-derived stem cells for wound healing. ACS Applied Materials & Interfaces. 2016;**8**(3):2423-2434. DOI: 10.1021/acsami.5b11811

[43] Chandika P, Ko SC, Jung WK. Marine-derived biological macromolecule-based biomaterials for wound healing and skin tissue regeneration. International Journal of Biological Macromolecules. 2015;**77**:24-35. DOI: 10.1016/j.ijbiomac.2015.02.050

[44] Lansdown AB. Calcium: A potential central regulator in wound healing in the skin. Wound Repair and Regeneration. 2002;**10**(5):271-285. DOI: 10.1046/j.1524-475X.2002.10502.x

[45] Merchant N, Smith K, Jeschke MG. An ounce of prevention saves tons of

lives: Infection in burns. Surgical Infections. 2015;**16**(4):380-387. DOI: 10.1089/sur.2013.135

[46] Norbury W, Herndon DN, Tanksley J, Jeschke MG, Finnerty CC. Infection in burns. Surgical Infections. 2016;**17**(2): 250-255. DOI: 10.1089/sur.2013.134

[47] Piacquadio D, Nelson DB. Alginates. A "new" dressing alternative. The Journal of Dermatologic Surgery and Oncology. 1992;**18**(11):992-995. DOI: 10.1111/j.1524-4725.1992.tb02773.x

[48] Wiegand C, Heinze T, Hipler UC. Comparative *in vitro* study on cytotoxicity, antimicrobial activity, and binding capacity for pathophysiological factors in chronic wounds of alginate and silver-containing alginate. Wound Repair and Regeneration. 2009;**17**(4): 511-521. DOI: 10.1111/j.1524-475X.2009.00503.x

[49] Poor AE, Ercan UK, Yost A, Brooks AD, Joshi SG. Control of multi-drug-resistant pathogens with non-thermal-plasma-treated alginate wound dressing. Surgical Infections. 2014; **15**(3):233-243. DOI: 10.1089/sur.2013.050

[50] Bystrom A, Claesson R, Sundqvist G. The antibacterial effect of camphorated paramonochlorophenol, camphorated phenol and calcium hydroxide in the treatment of infected root canals. Endodontics & Dental Traumatology. 1985;**1**:170-175. DOI: 10.1111/j.1600-9657.1985.tb00652.x

[51] Lee RM, Hartman PA, Stahr HM, Olson DG, Williams FD. Antibacterial mechanism of long-chain polyphosphates in Staphylococcus aureus. Journal of Food Protection. 1994;**57**:289-294. DOI: 10.4315/0362-028X-57.4.289

[52] Teixeira-da-Cunha MGA, Gomes RN, Roehrs N, Bozza FA, Prescott SM, Stafforini D, et al. Bacterial clearance is improved in septic mice by platelet-activating factor-acetylhydrolase (PAF-AH) administration. PLoS One. 2013;**8**: e74567. DOI: 10.1371/journal.pone.0074567

[53] Serbina NV, Jia T, Hohl TM, Pamer EG. Monocyte-mediated defense against microbial pathogens. Annual Review of Immunology. 2008;**26**:421-452. DOI: 10.1146/annurev.immunol.26.021607.090326

[54] Sjögren U, Figdor D, Spångberg L, Sundqvist G. The antimicrobial effect of calcium hydroxide as a short-term intracanal dressing. International Endodontic Journal. 1991;**24**:119-125. DOI: 10.1111/j.1365-2591.1991.tb00117.x

[55] Goh CH, Heng PW, Huang EP, Li BK, Chan LW. Interactions of antimicrobial compounds with cross-linking agents of alginate dressings. The Journal of Antimicrobial Chemotherapy. 2008;**62**:105-108. DOI: 10.1093/jac/dkn168

[56] Ngo DH, Kim SK. Sulfated polysaccharides as bioactive agents from marine algae. International Journal of Biological Macromolecules. 2013;**62**: 70-75. DOI: 10.1016/j.ijbiomac.2013.08.036

[57] Lee JB, Takeshita A, Hayashi K, Hayashi T. Structures and antiviral activities of polysaccharides from *Sargassum trichophyllum*. Carbohydrate Polymers. 2011;**86**:995-999. DOI: 10.1016/j.carbpol.2011.05.059

[58] Yan GL, Guo YM, Yuan JM, Liu D, Zhang BK. Sodium alginate oligosaccharides from brown algae inhibit Salmonella enteritidis colonization in broiler chickens. Poultry Science. 2011;**90**(7):1441-1448. DOI: 10.3382/ps.2011-01364

[59] Benavides S, Villalobos-Carvajal R, Reyes JE. Physical, mechanical and antibacterial properties of alginate film:

Effect of the crosslinking degree and oregano essential oil concentration. Journal of Food Engineering. 2012; **110**(2):232-239. DOI: 10.1016/j.jfoodeng.2011.05.023

[60] Khan S, Tøndervik A, Sletta H, Klinkenberg G, Emanuel C, Onsøyen E, et al. Overcoming drug resistance with alginate oligosaccharides able to potentiate the action of selected antibiotics. Antimicrobial Agents and Chemotherapy. 2012;**56**(10): 5134-5141. DOI: 10.1128/AAC.00525-12

[61] Pritchard MF, Powell LC, Menzies GE, Lewis PD, Hawkins K, Wright C, et al. A new class of safe oligosaccharide polymer therapy to modify the mucus barrier of chronic respiratory disease. Molecular Pharmaceutics. 2016;**13**(3):863-872. DOI: 10.1021/acs.molpharmaceut.5b00794

[62] Despond O, Proulx F, Carcillo JA, Lacroix J. Pediatric sepsis and multiple organ dysfunction syndrome. Current Opinion in Pediatrics. 2001;**13**:247-253. DOI: 10.1097/00008480-200106000-00006

[63] Gauglitz GG, Song J, Herndon DN, Finnerty CC, Boehning D, Barral JM, et al. Characterization of the inflammatory response during acute and post-acute phases after severe burn. Shock. 2008;**30**:503-507. DOI: 10.1016/j.jss.2007.12.440

[64] Finnerty CC, Przkora R, Herndon DN, Jeschke MG. Cytokine expression profile over time in burned mice. Cytokine. 2009;**45**:20-25. DOI: 10.1016/j.cyto.2008.10.005

[65] Finnerty CC, Herndon DN, Chinkes DL, Jeschke MG. Serum cytokine differences in severely burned children with and without sepsis. Shock. 2007;**27**: 4-9. DOI: 10.1097/01.shk.0000235138.20775.36

[66] Finnerty CC, Jeschke MG, Qian WJ, Kaushal A, Xiao W, Liu T, et al. Determination of burn patient outcome by large-scale quantitative discovery proteomics. Critical Care Medicine. 2013;**41**:1421-1434. DOI: 10.1097/CCM.0b013e31827c072e

[67] Chan G, Mooney DJ. Ca^{2+} released from calcium alginate gels can promote inflammatory responses *in vitro* and *in vivo*. Acta Biomaterialia. 2013;**9**: 9281-9291. DOI: 10.1016/j.actbio.2013.08.002

[68] Allantaz F, Chaussabel D, Banchereau J, Pascual V. Microarray-based identification of novel biomarkers in IL-1-mediated diseases. Current Opinion in Immunology. 2007;**19**(6): 623-632. DOI: 10.1016/j.coi.2007.10.003

[69] Dinarello CA. Biologic basis for interleukin-1 in disease. Blood. 1996; **87**(6):2095-2147. PMID: 8630372

[70] Echeverry S, Shi XQ, Haw A, Liu H, Zhang ZW, Zhang J. Transforming growth factor-beta1 impairs neuropathic pain through pleiotropic effects. Molecular Pain. 2009;**5**:16. DOI: 10.1186/1744-8069-5-16

[71] Zhu Y, Colak T, Shenoy M, Liu L, Mehta K, Pai R, et al. Transforming growth factor beta induces sensory neuronal hyperexcitability, and contributes to pancreatic pain and hyperalgesia in rats with chronic pancreatitis. Molecular Pain. 2012;**8**:65. DOI: 10.1186/1744-8069-8-65

[72] Panis C, Pavanelli WR. Cytokines as mediators of pain-related process in breast cancer. Mediators of Inflammation. 2015;**2015**:129034. DOI: 10.1155/2015/129034

[73] Lee WR, Park JH, Kim KH, Kim SJ, Park DH, Chae MH, et al. The biological effects of topical alginate treatment in an animal model of skin wound healing. Wound Repair and Regeneration. 2009;

17(4):505-510. DOI: 10.1111/j.1524-475X.2009.00496.x

[74] Lu Y, Huang CL, Yu F, Xu YJ. Effect of calcium alginate dressing on the cytokine contents, collagen synthesis - degradation balance and apoptosis gene expression in the wound after perianal abscess surgery. Journal of Hainan Medical University. 2017;**23**(18):65-68

[75] Iwamoto M, Kurachi M, Nakashima T, Kim D, Yamaguchi K, Oda T, et al. Structure–activity relationship of alginate oligosaccharides in the induction of cytokine production from RAW264. 7 cells. FEBS Letters. 2005; **579**:4423-4429. DOI: 10.1016/j.febslet.2005.07.007

[76] Ryan CA, Farmer EE. Oligosaccharide signals in plants: A current assessment. Annual Review of Plant Physiology and Plant Molecular Biology. 1991;**42**:651-674. DOI: 10.1146/annurev.pp.42.060191.003251

[77] Davis BK, Wen HT, Ting JPY. The Inflammasome NLRs in immunity, inflammation, and associated diseases. Annual Review of Immunology. 2011; **29**:707-735. DOI: 10.1146/annurev-immunol-031210-101405

[78] Murakami T, Ockinger J, Yu J, Byles V, McColl A, Hofer AM, et al. Critical role for calcium mobilization in activation of the NLRP3 inflammasome. Proceedings of the National Academy of Sciences of the United States of America. 2012;**109**(28):11282-11287. DOI: 10.1073/pnas.1117765109

[79] Zhou RB, Yazdi AS, Menu P, Tschopp J. A role for mitochondria in NLRP3 inflammasome activation. Nature. 2011;**469**(7354):221-225. DOI: 10.1038/nature09663

[80] Haug A, Myklastade S, Larsen B, Smidrod O. Correlation between chemical structure and physical properties of alginates. Acta Chemica Scandinavica. 1967;**21**:768-778. DOI: 10.3891/acta.chem.scand.21-0768

Chapter 2

A Study of the Use of Modified Collagen of Freshwater Fish as a Material for Personal Care Products

L.V. Antipova, S.A. Storublevtsev, S.A. Titov, S.S. Antipov, M.G. Khatkhokhu, M.S. Bolokov and V. V. Loboda

Abstract

The work is devoted to the use of collagen materials produced on the basis of connective tissues of hydrobionts. Their characteristics as potential means of personal hygiene and wound healing are investigated. The results of studies of physical and chemical characteristics of collagen materials from freshwater fish with a modified structure obtained in this paper indicate the prospects of their use as an absorbent layer of personal hygiene products, due to the high moisture absorption capacity, which is an order of magnitude higher than the moisture capacity of untreated collagen and higher moisture capacity of superadsorbing polymers required for use in personal hygiene products. The resulting material meets the requirements of sanitary and epidemiological safety, allergenic action on the skin, as can be concluded from the results of tests on animals, it does not. This material accelerates reparative processes to the same extent as collagen used in standard hemostatic sponges with the simplicity of its production technology, low cost, and availability of raw materials.

Keywords: hygiene, human, safety, hydration, moisture capacity, sorption capacity, deodorization, collagen, substances, fish raw materials

1. Introduction

Absorbing and deodorizing properties are especially important when improving and creating new medical means and materials, including those for individual use (personal hygiene).

Presently, the improvement of, for example, the napkins is focused primarily on the modification of their shape and design [1–3]; however, less attention is paid to a selection of moisture-absorbing layer materials for personal hygiene means, and their domestic production (in Russia) is absent. These materials can be divided now into three categories, i.e., the synthetics—for example, polyvinyl alcohols, polyethylene oxides, cross-linked polyacrylic esters [2]; natural materials—cellulose, guaric or xanthan gum; and modified natural materials—the cross-linked starches, sulphitic cellulose, Kraft cellulose [1]. The mixes of polymers of either synthetic or natural origin can be used. Particles of these polymers (they are called the superadsorbing polymers too) may have the form of powder, grains, granules, or fibers. Their use in the form of fibers is met more often because in this case the extensive capillary network is formed capable of binding a significant amount of moisture in macrocapillaries.

In case of choice of materials for functional layer, the preference, as we think, should be given to natural or modified natural materials. They do not, as a rule, cause allergy; they are environmentally friendly; and in general, they are perfectly recognized by the human body. Of all, collagen, particularly, the protein connecting tissues of animals, fish, and birds in whose organisms its content is the highest [4], belongs to natural materials, which could be used in personal hygiene.

At the same time, collagen is concentrated in the by-products and waste of the processing industries of agro-industrial complex [5] that are based on processing poultry, meat, and fish. In this regard, the sources of collagen can be considered as easily available and inexpensive, and their use for receiving collagenic substances decreases environmental pollution. The wide range of technological processing and a variety of sources [6–8] give the chance to use collagen not only as a part of the absorbing layers but also in other layers of personal hygiene. Collagen plays an important role in the implementation of reparative function of connecting tissue [9], it is fully compatible with human skin [10]; therefore, effects of irritation, discomfort, and other negative effects on skin may be expected as the system will be minimized.

Collagen is the fibrillary protein that forms fibrous materials [11–13], i.e., similar to cellulose, its fibers can form locks and gaps where water pours and remains entrapped. Moreover, like cellulose, collagen can swell and bulk up in water due to penetration of water into a structure of the material due to a large number of functional groups and their increased hydration ability [14, 15]. This property creates the prerequisites for use of collagen in the absorbing layers of personal hygiene means as the best material capable to compete with cellulose presently in use as well as other known materials.

Fish collagen in this regard is of the greatest interest, due to its special rheological characteristics facilitating the technological processing (its structure is low molecular in comparison with collagen of animals, it does not require obligatory hydrolysis when processing raw materials, and the final materials made of fish collagen are more elastic) [16]. However, the question of methods of its processing is open yet for saving and increasing its water-absorbing ability, and the question of sorption ability, especially to aromatic substances, and also its wound healing activity are not properly investigated yet.

The wide use of collagen in the cosmetic, medical, and food industries is interfered by its possible allergenicity. Thus, when holding mesotherapeutic procedures with collagen injections, allergic reaction develops in ~6% of women [17]. However, in this case, it must be taken into consideration that allergic effects are, as a rule, found in collagen of animal or sea fish origin. At the same time, for example in [18, 19], separate data are given that collagen of fresh-water fish shows minimum allergenicity or its total absence in comparison with collagen of sea fish. Yet, the results of both fresh-water fish collagen allergenicity research and its processing to increase its water-absorbing ability are unknown to the authors of this article. Moreover, there are but a few researches of microbiological and toxicological indicators of collagen of fish of internal natural reservoirs.

One more very interesting scope of collagen use is the creation of antidecubital bandages and sheets for people with limited mobility. High requirements of water-absorbing ability are obvious in this case. The hemostatic collagenic sponges are rather popular [20] having both styptic and aseptic effects and stimulating the processes of tissue regeneration. However, they are manufactured by way of hydrolysis of the collagen extracted by splitting cattle skin. The process of hydrolysis is extremely prolonged, and it demands the use of expensive reactants, which makes such sponges a very costly product. These shortcomings are eliminated in the products from fish collagen but the question of whether they will be able to compete with standard sponges' wound-healing properties requires a separate research.

The purpose of this work is to study the water-absorbing and sorption ability of collagen of fresh-water fish, search for opportunities of its increase, and assess the effect of a wound-healing, sanitary, and epidemiologic safety and allergenicity of the material received through collagen from fresh-water fish from internal natural basins of Russia.

2. Materials and methods

The objects of research were the collagenic product received by special processing of skins of pond fish using the author's technology (cf. the Russian Federation Patent No. 2614273). Skins of the silver carp were used, which is a valuable source of proteins among which the prevailing fraction is collagen [21]. Skins of fish were processed in weak solutions of alkalis and organic acids, and the received preparations were dried up with lyophilic process, in the course of which the material got a sponge form.

For the research of swelling capacity of the received material, the preset amount of water was used, and in our case, it was 20 ml, previously weighing the cup for processing and the studied material, measured the change of mass of water without sponge was measured when the constant volume of free liquid was eached, then the change of mass of a sponge was recalculated.

The research on the effect of a wound-healing property was made by histologic and histochemical methods [22] on animals of the same age received from a vivarium and the laboratories of the Voronezh State Medical University of N. N. Burdenko.

The first stage of research was carried out on animals and then on the human patient. All animals passed the quarantine, and they had no symptoms of diseases and received a standard diet. The average mass of an animal was 300 ± 25 g, and the dispersion of initial weight did not exceed 15%.

The research was made on 168 laboratory white rats divided into three groups: two of them are control and one is the main (see **Table 1**).

Wound modeling was carried out with the modified Sychennikov's technique (1974). Under ester anesthesia in aseptic conditions on the skin spot shaved from wool, after processing of skin with antiseptic solution, using the disposable medical scalpel a linear section of skin 1 cm long was made on the external surface of an average one-third of a hip, a fastion and the muscles. Soft tissues were clipped to extend the cut and warmed up. The area of wounds before an initiation of treatment in all groups averaged 26.0 ± 0.5 mm^2 without meaningful distinctions

Groups	Quantity of test animals	Group characteristics
No. 1, control	56	Without treatment
No. 2, control	56	Treatment with standard collagenic sponge
No.3, Tested species	56	Treatment with collagenic substance prepared from fish raw materials

Table 1.
Test group characteristics.

between the groups. The treatment of the second control group and the main group was applied right after the modeling of wounds.

In the first control group, the treatment was not used. In the second control group, the treatment of wound was made by washing it directly after modeling with 5 ml of 0.9% solution of sodium chloride and introduction into a wound of a standard collagenic sponge, which was cut out to fit the area of wound for its full closing. In the main group unlike the second control group used an analog of a standard sponge made of fish raw materials was used.

The dynamics of wound process arresting was estimated on the basis of the research methods listed below:

1. Clinical methods: the general condition of animals, indicators of a course of wound process (defect closing speed, exudation, presence of necrotic masses, emergence of granulations, epithelization, etc.).

2. Planimetric methods: the control of the area of a wound by the technique of Popova/the tsellofanografic method/and its dynamics. For calculation of percent of a daily change of the wound area, the following formula was used: $\% S = (S–Sn/S)*100\%$, where S is the area of a wound at the previous measurement; Sn is the area of a wound at the current measurement.

3. Histologic methods: to study the dynamics of histologic changes, the excision of tissue was made on the first, third, seventh, and eleventh day after the initiation of treatment with capture of an intact skin, a bottom and edge of a wound to a size 1.0 × 1.0 × 0.5 cm. The received material was fixed in the 10% solution of neutral formalin, dehydrated, further the 6 microns thick paraffin cuts were made and painted with hematoxylin-eosin and studied in a light microscope according to Van-Gizona. The images were obtained using the cross view of several fields of vision and analyzed in the image analysis system LeicaQwinStandartV2.6 (Leica, Germany), consisting of LeicaDRM microscope equipped with the “LeicaDC 300F” digital camera and a computer with the LeicaQ 550W software. Micrographs were processed using the Microsoft applications.

3. Histochemical methods

For histochemical research, the painted cuts of collagen samples were photographed at four hundredfold increase, and then contrasting of the reaction product was made equivalent to the histogram using the Threshold function filter allocation. For the allocated areas, the area in pixels was determined, which was recalculated in micrometers by the photograph with the same device with which the image was obtained, and the final object with an area of 1 micron was recalculated into pixels.

Investigation of the content of ribonucleic acid (RNA) with the technique with Azur V by Shea was made, which provided the selective identification of nucleatic and cytoplasmic RNA and made it possible to carry out the quantitative research of RNA content within the Malpighi sprout layer of epidermis.

Processing of cuts in 100% acetic anhydride at room temperature allowed to block the potentially reactive amino groups of protein, and the differentiation in tertiary butyl alcohol provided the removal of the molecules of Azur V that were not connected with RNA.

The content of sulph-hydrylic groups of proteins (SH group) was studied by Chevremont and Frederick’s method. This reaction represents the biochemical cysteine test at which the insoluble deposit of the Berlin azure is formed. Quantitative assessment of maintenance of SH-group within a Malpighi layer allowed to define the extent of maturing and the differentiation of epidermis at various methods of wound treatment.

Research of sanitary and epidemiologic safety was made at "The Center of Hygiene and Epidemiology in the Voronezh Region" Federal establishment (see the Test report No. 9627p of 09.02.2017). Determination of the content of heavy metals—arsenic, mercury, and lead—was made by GOST 26927-86, GOST 30178-96, and GOST 29188.2-9, and hydrogen indicator was measured according to GOST 26930-86. The skin-irritant effect of collagenic substances and its impact on mucous membranes were determined by the instruction 1.1.11-1352004, and the general toxic effect was determined by the alternative *in vitro* methods according to the document No. 29FTs1394 of January 29, 2002. Microbiological indicators were determined by the state standard specifications: (GOSTs) as follows: the total of mesophilic aerobic and facultative and aerobic microorganisms—by GOST ISO 21149-2013; *Candida albicans*—by GOST ISO 18416-2013; *Escherichia coli*—in accordance with GOST ISO 21150-2013; *Staphylococcus aureus*—in accordance with GOST ISO 22718-2013; and *Pseudomonas aeruginosa*—in accordance with GOST ISO 22717-2013.

The research of allergenicity was made in the same conditions (The Protocol on technical and toxicological research within the preclinical tests of porous medical materials from fish raw materials of July 01, 2014). Allergenic properties of collagenic substance of fish origin were studied on guinea pigs with skin applications.

Provocative skin tests were made as follows: before the applications, the sensitization of animals was made by repeated drawing of collagenic dispersion on skin. Daily applications were made on three guinea pigs with water dispersions of the modified collagen in cultivations on the cut-off site of skin, 1:1; 1:10 and 1:100, within 14 days (which corresponds to the duration of the incubatory period).

During the entire period of the experiment, the observed guinea pigs underwent measurement of body temperature, thickness of a skin fold on the place of application, and temperature on the place of introduction.

4. Results

The graphic dependences reflecting the kinetics of swelling capacity of collagen made of fish skin are presented in **Figure 1** (curve 1). The swelling capacity, i.e., the amount of water, absorbed by the unit of mass at hydration, is the characteristic that most adequately reflects the water-absorbing properties of the absorbing layer material of personal hygiene means.

In **Figure 1**, it is clear that the established value of swelling capacity of fish skin is approximately 3 g of moisture per 1 g of solid. After fish skin processing and receiving the material, its swelling capacity and, respectively, the moisture capacity increase approximately by 10 times (**Figure 1**, curve 2). At the same time, the amount of moisture bound with the sample is equal to 30 g per 1 g of solid. According to the data [2], the required value of this indicator for the superadsorbing polymer used in personal hygiene means is equal to 10 g of water per 1 g of solid. The processing we offered here allows to receive the material comparable or surpassing in moisture capacity of the polymers that are traditionally used in the absorbing layers of personal hygiene. Producing the collagenic materials from skin of fresh-water fish by modification is expedient because it allows to increase a material's moisture capacity.

The results of histologic analysis of experimental animals in the wound healing research are the following:

One day after the initiation of treatment: In all groups, the skin around the wounds was edematous and hyperemic; the palpation in the projection of a wound caused anxiety in an animal. The serous and hemorrhagic discharge was noted. In the groups where the collagenic sponges and collagenic substance from fish raw materials were used (the second control group and the main group), less expressed inflammatory reaction was noted visually (i.e., the reduction of hypostasis and hyperemia).

In the first control group, the histologic picture of a traumatic inflammation came to light: an injury of epidermis, hemorrhage, necrotic masses, or infiltration of a significant amount of neutrophilic leukocytes. Muscle fibers were displaced owing to intermuscular hypostasis. Connective tissue was inflamed. Hypostasis of tissue increased in paravual tissue and was followed by a compression of capillaries and venules, interfering with the blood outflow. The increased permeability of the vascular wall with an exit in tissue of forming elements and proteinaceous components of blood was observed. The most intensive basophyly in the RNA identification was observed within the basal and spike layers that indirectly indicate the most active metabolic processes at this level. The product of reaction (RNA) was sedimented in the cells of epidermis in the form of a disperse basophyly in cytoplasm, and the cells with larger granules were found.

In the second control group, the defect of epidermis was infiltrated densely with polymorphonuclear leukocytes, lymphocytes, plasmocytes, and macrophages. The expressed plethora and swelling of collagenic fibers were observed. Muscle fibers were moved apart owing to hypostasis, and some of them had signs of expressed dystrophy and phenomena of myolysis. In intermuscular spaces, the inflammatory infiltration was observed, expressed mainly with polymorphonuclear leukocytes.

In the main group in the area of the wound inflammatory reaction, moderate necrosis and hypostasis of soft tissue with leucocyte infiltration were observed.

Three days after the initiation of treatment: The behavior of experimental animals practically did not differ from the behavior of healthy species.

In the first control group, moderate inflammatory and edematous reactions of surrounding tissue were observed, which were less expressed in comparison with the first days. Inflammatory infiltrate contained cellular components: leukocytes

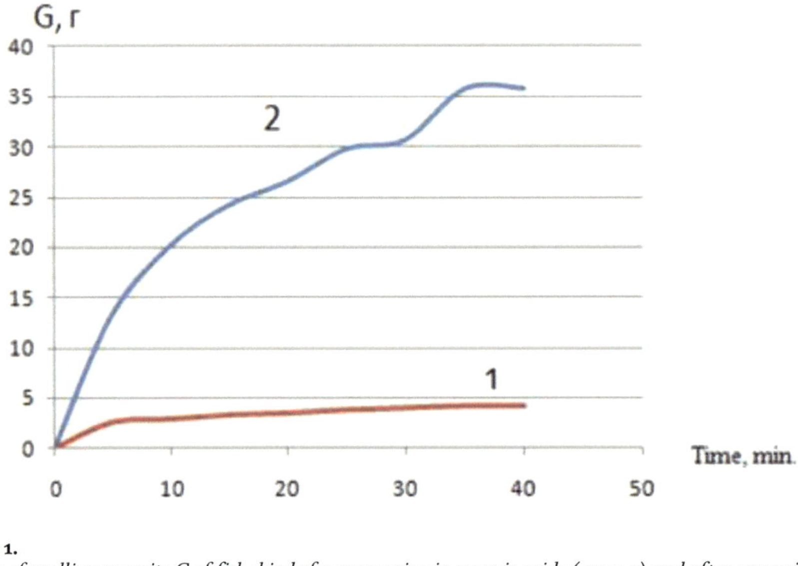

Figure 1.
Kinetics of swelling capacity G of fish skin before processing in organic acids (curve 1) and after processing (curve 2).

with decaying kernels and isolated tissue basophiles, macrophages, and lymphocytes; muscle fibers in the periphery of infiltrate had extended necrosis sites; single fibroblasts were visible; and in the wound, bottom isolated centers of granulated tissue were observed. Loss of fibrin was noted, which was connected with the walls of the wound defect. Insignificant amount of isolated collagenic fibers was observed in the mesh dermic layer. The intensity of epithelial cell coloring increased, especially in the deep layers of epidermis where uniform adjournment of basophile material or its localization in a perinuclear zone was observed.

In the second control group, moderate inflammatory and edematous reaction in a paravualny zone was observed, and granulation tissue and vascular and capillary network was formed on the surface, containing the visible organized (regular) fibrin, fibroblasts, histiocytes, and endoteliocytes, small congestions of polymorphic-nuclear leukocytes.

In the main group, the defect of epidermis was reduced, and edges of the wound were edematous. Restoration of skin integrity was observed, which was seen in the thickening of regional epidermis as a result of activation of reparative regeneration. The divergence of muscle fibers was noted due to the inflammatory infiltration filling the intermuscular spaces, and young granulations were formed in the periphery of the wound, which was the proliferative reaction of epidermis and skin elements. Collagenic fibers contained numerous infiltrated macrophages, fibroblasts, and eosinophilic leukocytes.

Seven days after the initiation of treatment: In the first control group, inflammatory reaction became less expressed, and infiltration with inflammation cells remained. The surface of the wound was filled with granulation tissue, and microabscesses of various localizations came to light. In the hem formation area, the increased quantity of fibroblasts, collagenic fibers wavy with the primary horizontal direction, and small capillaries in the formation phase were observed.

In the second control group, minimum signs of inflammatory reaction were observed, and in some wounds, there were leukocytes still, together with the expressed collagenic and angiogenesis. The surface of the wound was covered with epidermis with underlying granulation tissue enriched with completely filled blood vessels and capillaries, with a large number of eosinophils, fibroblasts, histiocytes and tissue basophiles, and a significant amount of collagenic fibers. On the periphery, there were the corpulent cells. In the depth of the wound, in intermuscular spaces, there was the formation of small capillaries.

In the main group, the restoration of tissue in a zone of wound defect was observed, and in the dermic layer, there were the well-formed collagenic fibers and granulation tissue.

Eleven days after the initiation of treatment: By the eleventh day, a hem had been formed completely in all groups, and the newly formed granulation tissue was clinically observed, which completely covered the wound.

In the second control group, the new epithelized hem was formed.

In the main group, the wound closed completely, and in the dermic layer, new collagenic fibers had been formed.

The wound area of all animals decreased in the main group, and in the second control groups, it was quicker, compared to that in the first control group (see **Table 2**).

Proceeding from clinical signs (**Table 3**), it is possible to conclude that after the initiation of treatment by the second day in the second control group and in the main group, and by the third day in the first control group, complete cut off of inflammation signs was noted with healing of wounds under a scab strip. It should be noted that the signs of inflammation or the first phase of wound process was stopped in the main group on average for 34–65% earlier compared to the first control group.

Animal groups	Initial wound size (area)	Time elapsed after wounds modeling, days			
		1	3	7	11
1 control group	26,1±0,5	18,5±0,5[1]	9,2±0,4[1]	4,5±0,4[1]	Well-
2 control group	26,0±0,5	12,8±0,6[1,2]	5,7±0,3[1,2]	1,5±0,3[1,2]	formed
the main group	26,1±0,5	12,6±0,6[1,2]	5,8±0,3[1,2]	1,5±0,3[1,2]	hem

[1]*Reliability of the distinctions in comparison with basic data;*
[2]*Reliability of distinctions in comparison with data of the 1st control group.*

Table 2.
Wound area change dynamics, for animals, mm^2.

Clinical signs	Groups		
	1 control	2 control	the main
Cut off of skin hyperaemia	1,8±0,5	1,3±0,5	1,3±0,4
Cut off of tissue hypostasis	2,2±0,3	1,7±0,4	1,6±0,3 *
Reduction of the quantity of separation to minimum	2,7±0,4	1,7±0,4 *	1,7±0,4 *

**Reliability of distinctions in comparison with 1-control group $r < 0.05$.*

Table 3.
Clinical signs of a course of wound process, days.

Groups	Content of ribonucleic acid (RNA)				Maintenance of SH-group			
Time, days	1	3	7	11	1	3	7	11
1 control	0,25	0,25	0,31	0,30	0,25	0,26	0,30	0,29
2 control		0,27	0,30	0,30		0,27	0,29	0,28
The main	0,28	0,29		0,31	0,31	0,29		0,30

Table 4.
Histochemical indicators of wound process.

Histochemical indicators of wound process are shown in **Table 4**, which shows that in all stages of its healing in the main group, the RNA level and SH-group are higher than in the first and second control groups. It prompts the actively going metabolic processes and approximately high rates of maturing and differentiation of epidermis.

When comparing the morphology of wounds, more expressed positive dynamics of healing of wounds in the second control and main groups is noted, revealed by the earlier decrease in tissue puffiness, organization of fibrin, and formation of collagen. It is established that the collagenic material imposed on a wound surface promoted local hemostatic action.

The analysis of toxicity of active ingredients showed that the acute state is not revealed in the experiment. Deviations of frequency of respiratory movements and warm reductions were within the norm regardless of the group of animals. Body temperature varied within ±0.7–0.8°C regardless also of the group of animals. The neurologic and behavioral status did not change. The total "Open field" test was 52.4 s, and the gravity 'sagging' test was 11.2 s. The qualitative analysis of immunoglobulin E showed the lack of sensibilization effect on the seventh day of the experiment.

Thus, during the course of the experimental study of the wound healing process, no distinctions were found between the application of a standard collagenic sponge and collagenic substance from fish raw material. In comparison with the control group of the animals who did not receive additional treatment the data confirming the acceleration of reparative processes in soft tissue under the influence of a standard collagenic sponge and collagenic substance from the fish raw materials which are especially expressed in the first phase of wound healing process that was shown in the stimulation of a collagenic genesis, activation of the metabolic processes which are followed by the increased level of reactions of RNA and SH-group identification. The conducted pilot studies did not reveal toxic and allergic effects of collagenic substance made of fish raw material both in the analysis of clinical data and when studying the results of histologic and histochemical analysis.

The results of the research of sanitary and hygienic safety of collagenic substance made of fish collagen are shown in **Table 5**, which goes to show that deviations from safety standards were not revealed.

In the allergenicity tests during the entire period of the experiment, there were no changes in the clinical status of animals and no changes in the skin condition over the area of collagenic substance applications. Based on the received results, the response on allergenicity was estimated negatively.

The main mechanism of influence of collagen is the implementation of reparative function of connecting tissue. Introduction of collagen-based composition of medicines promotes the extension of the medicines' effect due to high osmotic activity providing the dehydrating action on a tissue in the inflammation. Such medicines can be used as an effective wound covering [7]. The napkins based on collagen impregnated with antibiotics have good compatibility with skin tissue, thanks to low allergenicity and biodestruction of collagen. For example, the best results of surgical treatment were received for the approbation in Maykop, the Republic of Adygea, at the Adygeian Republican Clinical Hospital. During the tests, 10 patients with different diagnoses were observed, i.e., acute paraproctitis, acute osteomyelitis, postoperative hems, burns, and trophic ulcers. When imposing

No.	The defined indicators	Analysis results	Size of admissible level	Units of measurements
1	Arsenic	less than 0,025	below 5,0	mg/kg
2	Mercury	less than 0,03	below 1,0	mg/kg
3	Lead	less than 0,25	below 5,0	mg/kg
4	Hydrogen indicator	4,6	2,5-8,5	-
5	Skin irritant action	0 (not found)	0 (not found)	points
6	Impact on mucous membranes (once)	0 (not found)	0 (not found)	points
7	The all-toxic action determined by the alternative in vitro methods	absent	absent	-
8	Total of mesophilic aerobic and facultative and aerobic microorganisms	85	Less than 10^{-3}	
9	Candida albicans	no	not allowed	-
10	Escherichia coli	no	not allowed	-
11	Staphilococcus aureus	no	not allowed	-
12	Pseudomonas aeruginosa	no	not allowed	-

Table 5.
Results of tests of the modified collagen for sanitary and hygienic safety.

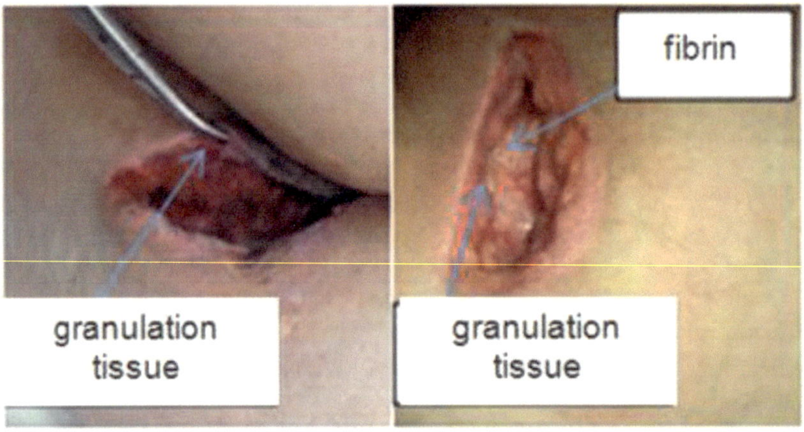

Figure 2.
Dynamics of treatment with application of collagen-based napkins (3 days): (a) result before use of collagen; (b) result after use.

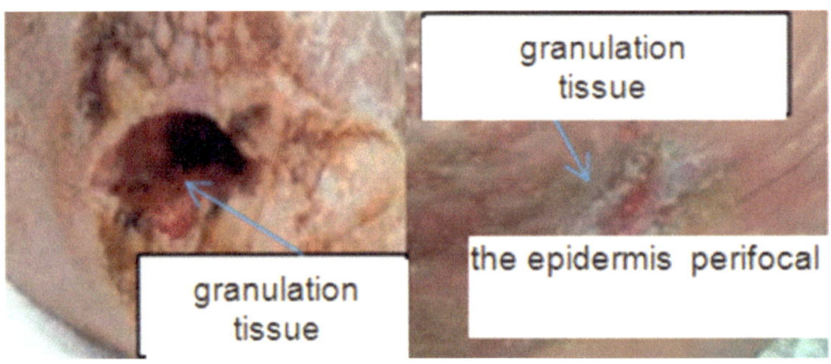

Figure 3.
Dynamics of treatment with collagen-based wipes (3 days): (a) the result before the collagen application; (b) the result after the application of collagen.

a collagen-based napkin as a bandage to patients with a sharp paraproctitis, the satisfactory condition of the patient, without therapeutic side effects, the lack of necrosis, and the formation of granulation tissue, with positive wound healing results (**Figure 2**), were observed.

Collagen-based napkins were applied on the acute osteomyelitis wounds, which arose after foot amputation (on the lower extremity, see **Figure 3**). The results are positive, viz., the patient's satisfactory dynamics without therapeutic side effects and stable formation of granulation tissue were observed.

Collagen film covering was applied for the treatment of postoperative hems. The results are positive, viz., the patient's satisfactory dynamics without therapeutic side effects and stable formation of granulation tissue and wound healing were observed on the fifth day. Film application is shown in **Figure 4**.

The offered covering allows the wounds, burns, and ulcers to be treated well and quickly, and it can be used for treatment of the bleeding traumatic damages, flat granulating slow wounds to a stage of regeneration, trophic ulcers, decubituses, and when healing donor sources. The of wound healing films demonstrate the stabilizing properties that remain reliable for a rather long time. Results of healing on the sixth day with the use of the collagen-based materials of fish origin are shown in **Table 6**.

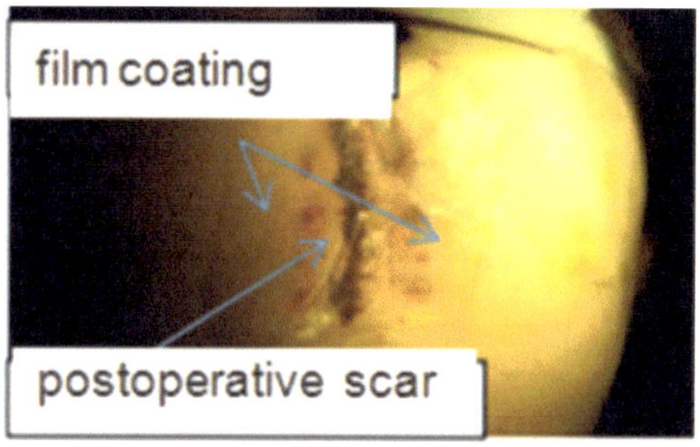

Figure 4.
Application of a collagen film.

Patient	Wound area (cm)	Wound size 1st day	Wound size 2nd day	Wound size 3rd day	Wound size 4th day		Wound size 5th day	Wound size 6th day
№1 Chronic osteomielitis)	5×3×3	5×3×3	4,5×2,5×3	4,5×2,5×2,5	4×2×2,5		4×2×2	2,5×1×1
№2 Acute paraproctitis)	9×5×5	9×5×5	8,5×4,5×4,5	8,5×4×4	8×4×4		7,5×3×3	6,5×2,5×2,5
№3 Acute paraproctitis)	7×4×4	7×3,5×4	7×3×3,5	6,5×3×3,5	6,5×3×3		6×3×3	6×2,5×2,5
№4 ECH without abscellation	13	Hem reddened	Hem reddened		Restoration, reddened			Complete restoration

Table 6.
Results of healing for the 6th day.

5. Discussion

Processing of biopolymers in organic acids is quite often applied for the purpose of modification of biomacromolecules and adding to a material the necessary physical and chemical properties [23–25]. There are also mentions of processing of fish collagen organic acids for simplification of its dispergating [26, 27]. It is possible due to the processes of destruction of fibers of collagen [28] beginning when the processing in acids starts, apparently, it is connected with a rupture of communications between polypeptide chains of collagen. As a result of change of structure, the extensive capillary network where moisture is caught increases the general moisture capacity of the studied material.

Identical wound healing action of a standard collagenic sponge based on modified fish collagen can be explained as follows:

The molecule of collagen of mammals consists of three polypeptide α-chains, mutually coiled in a structure of the threefold right twirled superspiral like a three-vein rope [11] that gives this structure high durability and big molecular weight. These chains are connected among themselves by cross links. Distinctive features of fish collagen are the 'single-coil' structure and the parallel arrangement of polypeptide chains, in which molecular mass is much lower than of collagen of mammals and it is preserved at the level of a tropocollagen [19]. As a result, fish collagen is not strong enough, and the collagen of mammals is possibly not so strongly connected with other elements of tissue. Therefore, fish collagen does not require preliminary hydrolysis, and when processed in weak alkaline and acid solutions, it is allocated easily from fish skins. Then, when in contact with the wound surface, the polypeptide chains of fish collagen are built into a structure of a regenerate, similar to the fragments of a molecule of animal collagen after its long hydrolysis in the rigid modes.

From the submitted data on a sanitary and epidemiologic condition of examinees of samples it follows that the studied collagenic substance, contains ions of heavy metals in concentration tens times less than the admissible level, it does not render the skin irritating and all-toxic action, and an effect on mucous membranes, and moreover it contains much smaller amounts of mesophilic aerobic and facultative and aerobic microorganisms below the admissible threshold. In the studied samples, there were no pathogenic microflora at all. Thus, the obtained collagenic materials of fish origin are biologically safe, they have an expressed effect on wound healing, and the technology of their preparation differs favorably from the process of production of standard materials.

Except the excellent moisture-absorbing and wound-healing properties, the modified fish collagen has the essential occluding ability. Thus, in [29, 30], the high sorption capacity of fish collagenic substances have been proven due to the presence of various functional groups, hydrophilic and hydrophobic sites, in a molecule structure. This fact allows to assess positively the prospects of collagenic substances' use as a part of personal hygiene means with a deodorizing effect.

6. Conclusion

The results of research of physical and chemical characteristics of collagenic materials received in the real work from fresh-water fish with the modified structure testify to prospects of their use as the absorbing layer of personal hygiene means, in view of the high moisture-absorbing ability which is 10 times higher than a moisture capacity of the raw collagen and is higher than the moisture capacity of the super-adsorbing polymers demanded for use in personal hygiene means. The material thus obtained conforms to the requirements of sanitary and epidemiologic safety, allergenic action of skin as it is possible to conclude by results of tests on animals, it does not render. This material accelerates the reparative processes as much as the collagen used in standard hemostatic sponges, having the simplicity of technology of its production, low cost, and availability of raw materials. These results altogether give the grounds for perspective considerable development of domestic production of fish collagenic materials including their use as a part of personal hygiene means and surgery.

New environmentally friendly sources for production of collagen—an urgent scientific and technical problem of the present as it is popular and proved **conclusions** in biomedical technologies, structure of specialized food for rehabilitation and during the post-operational and post-traumatic periods. It has an extraordinary demand in cosmetology for the production of cosmetics of various functionalities: as a part of shampoos, creams, etc.; for restoration and improvement of structure of hair; increase in their volume; and rejuvenation of skin. The research of properties and the characteristic of unique biopolymers of the collagenic nature shall give way to operate respective technologies in the production of food, cosmetics, and medical products and medicines; to extend this segment and to stabilize the situation of Russia in the international market; and to expand the range and scopes of products of cutting of fish. Thus, it is possible to claim that production of collagen from collateral fish raw materials answers the principles of rational environmental management and, at last, it is economic.

Its application is competitive and perspective both in its original form and for the production of foodstuff, medical supplies, and cosmetics in the internal and world markets.

Author details

L.V. Antipova[1*], S.A. Storublevtsev[1], S.A. Titov[2], S.S. Antipov[3,4,5†], M.G. Khatkhokhu[2], M.S. Bolokov[6] and V.V. Loboda[6]

1 Voronezh State University of Engineering Technologies, Voronezh, Russia

2 Maikop State Technological University, Maikop, Russia

3 School of Life Sciences, Immanuel Kant Baltic Federal University, Kaliningrad, Russia

4 Voronezh State University, Voronezh, Russia

5 Institute of Cell Biophysics RAS, Pushchino, Russia

6 Maikop City Hospital of Adygea Republic, Maikop, Russia

† S.S. Antipov was supported by the Russian Academic Excellence Project at the Immanuel Kant Baltic Federal University.

*Address all correspondence to: antipova.l54@yandex.ru

References

[1] Kessler T et al. Absogbing product hygienic gasket. Patent US No. 2229868; 2004

[2] Mason PC et al. Inserting gasket with the indicator of improved characteristics. Patent US No. 2373911; 2007

[3] Paukshto MV et al. Collagen materials, films and methods of their production. Patent US No. 2009125186/05; 2007

[4] Antipova LV. The Collagens: Sources, Properties, Applications. Voronezh; 2014. (in Russian)

[5] Glotova IA, Boltachev V. Rheological characteristics of multifunctional disperse systems based on collagen proteins of animal tissues. Advances in Modern Natural Science. 2008;**2**:43-44. (in Russian)

[6] Batechko SA. Collagen. A New Strategy of Preservation of Health and Youth. Koleczkowo; 2010

[7] Istranova EV, Istranov LP, Tchaikovsky EA. Collagen modification: Physico-chemical and pharmaceutical properties and applications. Chemical and Pharmaceutical Journal. 2006;**40**(2):32-36. (in Russian)

[8] Antipova LV, Storublevtsev SA, Bobreshova MV. Skins of fish—As an object for obtaining collagen substances. In: Scientific Conference "Science, Technology and Technology" Plovdiv LIX; 2012. pp. 976-978. (in Russian)

[9] Antipova LV, Korobleva SA, Bolgova SB. Prospects of obtaining and application for wound healing materials based on collagen fish. In: Proceedings of the 1st International Congress of Industrial and Scientific Networks in Cooperation with Pharmaceutical, Chemical and Food Industries; Voronezh; 2014. pp. 116-120. (in Russian)

[10] Ignatieva NY. Collagen - the basic protein of connective tissue. Aesthetic Medicine Journal. 2005;**3**(4):257-258. (in Russian)

[11] Boriskina EP. Physical Factors of Stability of Three-Spiral Collagen-Type. Kharkiv; 2006. (in Ukraine)

[12] Vasiliev MP. Collagen Filaments, Fibrous and Film Materials. St. Petersburg; 2004. (in Russian)

[13] Gabuda SP, Gaidash AA. The structure of collagen and disorder of the water subsystems in fibrillar proteins. Biofizika. 2005;**2**:231-235. (in Russian)

[14] Li GY. Physicochemical properties of collagen isolated from calf limed splits. Journal of American Leather Chemists Association. 2003;**98**:224-229

[15] Finkelstein AV, Ptitsin OB. Physics of Protein. KDU; 2012

[16] Bechir A, Sirbu R, Leca M, Maris M, Maris DA, Cadar E. The nanobiotechnology of obtaining of collagen gels from Marin fish skin and yours reological properties for using like new materials in dental. International Journal of Medical, Health, Biomedical, Bioengineering and Pharmaceutical Engineering. 2008;**2**(6):190-196

[17] Kazimirova K. Unidentified collagen. Cosmetology. 2012;**6**:90-93

[18] Dvoryaninova OP. Biotechnological potential of internal fish water bodies [Dr. Tech. Sci. Diss]. Voronezh; 2013. (in Russian)

[19] Dvoryaninova OP. Production, properties and application of collagen dispersion of fish skin [Dr. Tech. Sci. Diss]. Voronezh; 2002. (in Russian)

[20] Istranov LP, Aboyants RK, Istranova YV. Antimicrobial hemostatic

sponge. Patent of the Russian Federation No. 2396984; Dated March 27, 2010

[21] Spiridonova MV, Dvoryaninova OP, Sokolov AV. Products of carp cutting—As a source of protein in the technology of forage production. International Student Scientific Bulletin. 2016;**3**:136-137. (in Russian)

[22] Alekseeva NT. Morphological evaluation of regenerate during healing of purulent skin wounds under the influence of various methods of regional exposure. Journal of Anatomy and Histopathology. 2014;**3**(2):14-18

[23] Matthews JA. Biomacromolecules. 2002;**3**:232-238

[24] Bhattarai N. Biomaterials. 2005;**3**(26):6176-6184

[25] Mo X, Chen Z, Weber HJ. Electrospun nanofibres of collagen - chitosan and p(LLA-CL) for tissue engineering. Frontiers of Medicine - Science in China. 2007;**1**(1):20-23

[26] Semenycheva LV. Method for producing acetic dispersion of high-molecular fish collagen. Patent RF No. 2567171; 2015. (in Russian)

[27] Vorobyov VI. Use of fish collagen and products of its hydrolysis. In: Proceedings of the Kaliningrad state technical University; Vol. 13; 2008. pp. 55-58. (in Russian)

[28] Glotova IA, Ryazhskikh VI, Galochkina NA, Makarkina EN, Galochkin MN. Production of functional disperse systems based on collagen proteins: formalized approach to the description of heat and mass transfer processes. Basic Research Journals. 2012;**11**:383-388. (in Russian)

[29] Antipova LV, Storublevtsev SA. Sorption properties of collagen substances in the creation of meat functional foods. In: International Scientific and Practical Conference Dedicated to the Memory of Vasily Gorbatov; Vol. 1; 2016. pp. 367-369. (in Russian)

[30] Storublevtsev SA, Antipova LV, Stukalo OG, Bolgova SB. Evaluation of bacteriostatic effect of immobilized on collagen carrier of antibiotics and silver ions in providing asepsis. Hygiene and Sanitation. 2015;**9**(94): 54-57. (in Russian)

Chapter 3

Plant Macromolecules as Biomaterials for Wound Healing

Felipe Domingos de Sousa, Francisco Rogênio da Silva Mendes, Jose Jovanny Bermudez-Sierra, Ayrles Fernanda Brandão da Silva, Mirele da Silveira Vasconcelos, Tamiris de Fátima Goebel de Souza, Marília de Oliveira Nunes, Antônio Eufrásio Vieira-Neto, Marcos Roberto Lourenzoni, Rosueti Diógenes de Oliveira-Filho, Adriana Rolim Campos, Renato de Azevedo Moreira and Ana Cristina de Oliveira Monteiro-Moreira

Abstract

Natural biomolecules are increasingly relevant for biomedical applications and tissue engineering for being able to produce an effect on chemical signals, organization of cells, and restitution of extracellular matrix in lesioned tissues. In this chapter, we will address the potential of plant macromolecules, in particular, carbohydrates and proteins such as hemicelluloses and lectins. While lectins are mostly carbohydrate-binding proteins, which can interact with cell surfaces to initiate anti-inflammatory pathways, as well as immunomodulatory functions, hemicelluloses are remarkably known by their ability to form viscous solutions even at low concentrations, which makes them an excellent candidate as vehicle to carry different sorts of biomolecules. Taking into account the complexity of the whole healing process, as an overlapping and coordinated cascade of events, most of the properties presented here by those materials may be of interest to the wound-care market.

Keywords: lectins, galactomannans, biomolecules, polysaccharides

1. Introduction

Skin is the largest organ, which presents a fairly robust arrangement, working as a natural shield against physical, chemical, and bacterial damage to the body. When it suffers any disruption in this arrangement by means of acute lesions, the skin goes through a fascinating repair process finalizing in wound closure and leaving some scars. This complex mechanism is dependent on many cell types and mediators

IntechOpen

interacting to maintain the physiological regulation of skin [1, 2]. Chronic wound results in situations such as diabetes or vascular lesions, when defective skin usually persists causing the loss of integrity, and in some cases, the overlapping of structural layers, as well as delayed skin tissue recovery [3].

Human body tissues present a wide range of physical characteristics, which include stiffness and porosity. A multidisciplinary interface between areas such as cell biology, biotechnology, mechanics, materials science, bioengineering, and clinical research has been used to contribute significantly to tissue engineering. Many wound dressings have been developed seeking to restore and improve tissue function by generating new biocompatible substitutes or by rebuilding these tissues [4, 5]. However, these sorts of materials are quite costly, which might affect the widespread adoption.

From this perspective, an ideal wound dressing would maintain a microenvironment in the injured bed and would direct the specific healing properties for each type of wound or disease that affects the patient under treatment. The dressing should also keep the moisture balance, which works as a barrier of protection against infections and would provide thermal insulation for the wound [6]. Therefore, recent technologies for biomedical applications invest in the development of scaffolds able to mimic the natural environment for skin grown and regeneration after damage [4].

Polysaccharide-based biomaterials emerge in the field of tissue engineering, as they are mainly used as hydrogels for the effective treatment of wounds and skin burns. They can be categorized as neutral (e.g., glucans, dextran, and cellulose), acids (acid hyaluronic), basic (chitosan) or sulfated polysaccharides (heparin and chondroitin). The most popular and naturally produced biomaterials of polysaccharide origin are chitosan, hyaluronic acid, and alginate. These polysaccharides may also be subdivided into homopolysaccharides such as glucans, cellulose, dextran and chitosan, and heteropolysaccharides such as alginates, agarose, carrageenan, pectin, galactomannans and xyloglucans. All exhibit peculiar physicochemical properties and a considerable biocompatibility and biodegradability, and thus have important applications in biomedical fields [4].

In this chapter, we focus our attention to plant macromolecules such as carbohydrates and proteins (in particular hemicelluloses and lectins) as biomolecules for wound healing applications.

2. Wound healing

Wound healing is a critical, complex and highly coordinated process to maintain skin function. Immediately after injury, a multitude of molecular and cellular systems are activated to suspend blood loss, eliminate microorganisms and foreign materials, and recompose injured tissue [3]. These cellular and biochemical events in wound repair can be divided into the following steps: hemostasis, inflammatory response, cell proliferation and synthesis of the elements that make up the extracellular matrix (ECM), and the later period, called remodeling. These stages are not mutually exclusive but overlapping over time [7].

In physiological conditions, platelets circulate in the vicinity of the vascular walls and are activated when the continuity of the endothelial layer is ruptured and the underlying subendothelial matrix is exposed, initiating the first stage of tissue repair, characterized by hemostasis and the formation of a matrix in the wound bed. This matrix is the result of the adhesion and aggregation of circulating platelets to the components of the underlying ECM. Damaged tissue and aggregated platelets trigger extrinsic and intrinsic coagulation pathways to stabilize the fibrin platelet clot. This whole process forms a framework for the migration and proliferation of other cells involved in wound healing, as well as a reservoir for cytokines and growth factors [8].

The inflammatory phase then begins as an innate immune response to promote the elimination of cellular and extracellular debris as well as pathogenic microorganisms. Both platelets and leukocytes release inflammatory cytokines providing a chemotactic gradient for additional leukocytes to be attracted and potentiate the inflammatory process. Among the inflammatory factors are interleukin IL-1α, IL-1β, IL-6, IL-8, tumor necrosis factor (TNF-α), platelet-derived growth factor (PDGF) and transforming growth factor-β. Clearly, PDGF plays an important role early in the chemotaxis of neutrophils, monocytes, smooth muscle cells and fibroblasts, while TGF-β stimulates cytokine secretion from macrophages and enhances chemotaxis of fibroblasts and smooth muscle cells [9].

The initial leukocyte response is dominated by neutrophils in the first 2–5 days, with macrophages taking over from the third day. Neutrophils have three main functions. First, they generate free radicals via the myeloperoxidase pathway to kill bacteria, an important action for healing because wounds that have bacterial infection will not heal normally. They also debride the wound through the secretion of specific proteolytic enzymes that break non-viable tissue, such as serine proteases and matrix metalloproteinase (MMP-2 and -9). Hence, the neutrophils phagocyte the dead bacteria and the remained matrix. They usually undergo apoptosis when their tasks are completed and are cleansed by macrophages [9, 10].

The monocytes begin to migrate to the wound and mature into macrophages. They become the most important regulatory cell in the inflammatory reaction. In the early stages of inflammation, M1 phenotype macrophages are associated with the phagocytic activity of remaining bacteria, sequestration and production of pro-inflammatory mediators. After this period, M1 becomes the subset M2, revealing a reparative phenotype of macrophages [1]. M2 macrophages are involved in the synthesis of anti-inflammatory mediators and tissue cleansing. These cells remove obsolete neutrophils, non-functional host cells, damaged matrix, and foreign debris. M2 cells also secrete various cytokines, growth factors and other mediators, such as TGF-α, TGF-β, basic fibroblast growth factor (β-FGF), PDGF and vascular endothelial growth factor (VEGF) to amplify and resolve inflammation. At this stage of healing, macrophages regulate the proliferative stage by stimulating fibroblasts, keratinocytes and endothelial cells to differentiate, proliferate and migrate, leading to new ECM deposition, re-epithelialization and wound neovascularization [11].

The goal of the proliferative stage is to decrease the area of contracted tissue and fibroplasia, establishing a viable epithelial barrier to activate keratinocytes. TGF-β stimulated fibroblasts differentiate into myofibroblasts rich in alpha smooth muscle actin and can amplify pseudopodia, joining fibronectin and collagen in the ECM. This event provides wound contraction, which is important in the repair process, helping the edges of the wound approach. These cells are also producers of ECM substances (collagen, fibronectin, glycosaminoglycans, proteoglycans and hyaluronic acid), which interact with the cells to mediate migration, growth and differentiation. This stage is characterized by the lesion closure, which includes angiogenesis, fibroplasia and re-epithelialization [7, 12].

The final stage of wound healing is characterized by the development of new epithelium and formation of scar tissue, a process known as remodeling, which can last for a year or stay for a longer period. The main purpose of the remodeling step is to achieve maximum tensile strength through reorganization, degradation and resynthesis of ECM. Together with intracellular matrix maturation, collagen bundles increase in diameter, whereas hyaluronic acid and fibronectin are degraded. The force of traction of the wound progressively increases with the deposition of collagen, and these fibers can recover approximately 80% of the force compared to normal tissue, but the force of the original tissue can never be recovered again [12].

As demonstrated, many factors can alter positively or negatively the cell interactions and the signaling mechanisms during the wound healing process. Plant-derived compounds are among these factors and are able to improve the healing process through different mechanisms.

3. Plant-derived compounds

Medicinal plants have been extensively used worldwide as traditional treatment for various diseases due to being a source of phytochemicals, which are nonnutritive substances present in plants enhancing tissue regeneration and acting as pro-angiogenic agents for wound healing. In addition, bioactive products extracted from plants arouse scientific and commercial interests for the development of new drugs [13]. On the other hand, plants are also source of many macromolecules such as carbohydrate and proteins extensively used as biomaterials for wound healing applications.

3.1 Essential oils

Essential oils (EOs) are the largest group of secondary metabolites biosynthesized by plant as a complex of monoterpenes (10 carbons) and sesquiterpenes (15 carbons), mainly related to plant defense mechanisms. Also known as volatile oils or aromatic plant essences, they can be found in a multitude of plant tissues such as flowers, leaves, barks, etc. Obtained by aqueous extraction or steam distillation, or cold pressing in the case of citric fruits, they have been extensively employed in cosmeceuticals and dermaceutical products [14, 15].

In the healing process, the OEs stand out for their anti-inflammatory and antimicrobial properties. The efficacy in inhibiting bacterial development, including antibiotic-resistant strains, yeasts and filamentous fungi, has boosted the study of the antimicrobial activity of essential oils. Some oils extracted from medicinal plants demonstrated therapeutic potential in combating biofilms, a mechanism of virulence produced by pathogenic microorganisms, resistant to antibiotics [16]. Carvacrol and Thymol, for example, are monoterpenes widely found in essential oils *Origanum* genus, presenting antibacterial and antifungal activities [17] in addition to analgesic effect [18]. In several studies, it has been reported that interactions between the components of EOs, even in small concentrations, may lead to antagonistic, additive or synergistic effects [15].

Although EOs are a mix of plant molecules with many applications such as antimicrobial, anti-inflammatory, besides potential healing properties, as stated above, we draw our attention here to plant polysaccharides and lectins.

3.2 Carbohydrates

Essentially, seeds play an important role in the reproductive strategies of certain species and represent a critical phase in life cycle of plants. Also, they play a vital role in diet and human health, which fosters a wide range of potential applications explored by science and technology. Substantial contributions to human well-being and health have emerged from these applications in fields such as the development of biopharmaceuticals [19].

All cells in higher plants present in their cell wall a complex network formed by numerous polymers including cellulose, non-cellulosic polysaccharides (pectin), structural glycoproteins and, on the secondary wall, lignin. A singular characteristic of plant cell walls is the presence of cellulose, consisting of glucose chains linked to β-(1→4), organized in microfibrils [20, 21]. Intertwined with these microfibrils, a series of hemicelluloses, which are polysaccharides that have similar characteristics to cellulose, are found crosslinked to it.

3.2.1 Plant cell wall polysaccharides

Cell wall polysaccharides can be divided into structural and storage polysaccharides. Primary and secondary walls contain cellulose and hemicelluloses, pectin in addition to enzymes and structural proteins, while the secondary walls contain few proteins or pectin, but usually contain lignin. Secondary cell walls appear when the cell interrupts its growth and often exhibit elaborate specializations for which the incorporation of lignin is usually the most distinctive characteristic. Therefore, the secondary walls of cotyledonary and endospermic cells in seeds of many species do not have lignin and contain low cellulose [22, 23].

On the other hand, in some seeds, cell wall of storage tissues (endosperm or cotyledon) is quite thick and contains deposits of polysaccharides, which are mobilized after germination. These polysaccharides are called cell wall storage polysaccharides (CWSPs) and are split into: mannans; galactomannans and glucomannans; xyloglucans and galactans [22].

Storage polysaccharides are mostly water soluble and form viscous and stable dispersions, normally absorbing a large amount of this solvent. It assures water around the embryo during the imbibition and germination process, helping protect against dehydration [22].

3.2.1.1 Galactomannans

Galactomannans are neutral cell wall polysaccharides, commonly found in endosperm of dicotyledonous seeds. They perform the storage function, being usually catabolized to provide energy and carbon skeletons to the plant during germination. They are more abundant in seeds of *Leguminosae* family in which the four major sources of commercial importance are locust bean (*Ceratonia siliqua*), guar (*Cyamopsis tetragonoloba*), tara (*Caesalpinia spinosa* Kuntze) and fenugreek (*Trigonella foenum-graecum* L.) [24].

As can be seen in **Figure 1**, galactomannan are heterogeneous polysaccharides presenting a linear chain of D-mannopyranose residues linked by β-glycoside bonds (1→4) with D-galactopyranosyl attached to these via α-type glycosidic bonds (1→6). In spite of this structure, galactomannans are also called hemicelluloses,

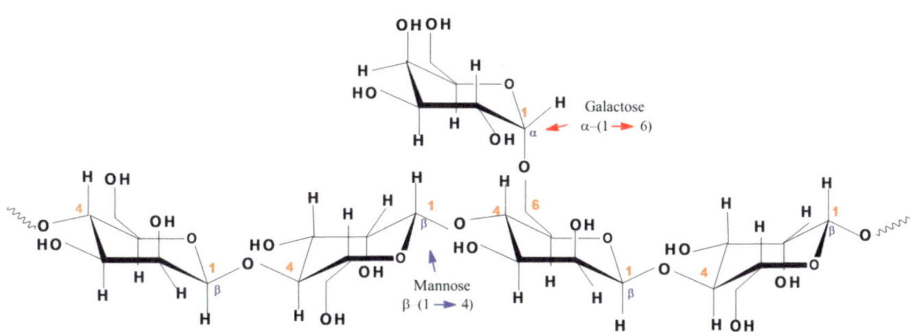

Figure 1.
General structure of galactomannan, considered a hemicellulose by sharing the equatorial β-(1→4)-linked backbone with cellulose. Galactosyl residues are attached to the main backbone by α-glycosyl bonds.

and variations in this Gal/Man ratio cause significant changes in physicochemical parameters such as average molecular weight, intrinsic viscosity and polydispersity of this natural polymers. In addition, the solubility in water is significantly affected by this sugar ratio, which may vary depending of source and isolation procedure. As observed, the higher is the main backbone substituted by galactosyl residues, the more is soluble the galactomannan in water [25].

3.2.1.2 Xyloglucans

Xyloglucans are plant polysaccharides with both structural and storage function, found in the primary cell wall of cotyledon of various seeds. Their main chain consists of D-glucopyranose linked by β-(1→4) and branched in O-6 by α-D-xylopyranoside units, which can also be substituted in O-2 by units of β-D-galactopyranosyl [22]. This group of polysaccharides plays a fundamental role controlling cell expansion. Experimental results evidenced xyloglucans associated with microfibrils, suggesting that like other hemicelluloses, they are able to provide mechanical resistance and physical integrity to the complex arrangements in plant cell walls [26].

With reference to this association to cellulose, xyloglucans are bound via hydrogen bonds and due to their long polysaccharide chains, they assure the maintenance of network microfibrils in cell wall expansion [22]. **Figure 2** displays the common structure of storage xyloglucans, which make them able to form hydrogels and films solutions to be molded in wound dressings able to carrier potential healing molecules [27].

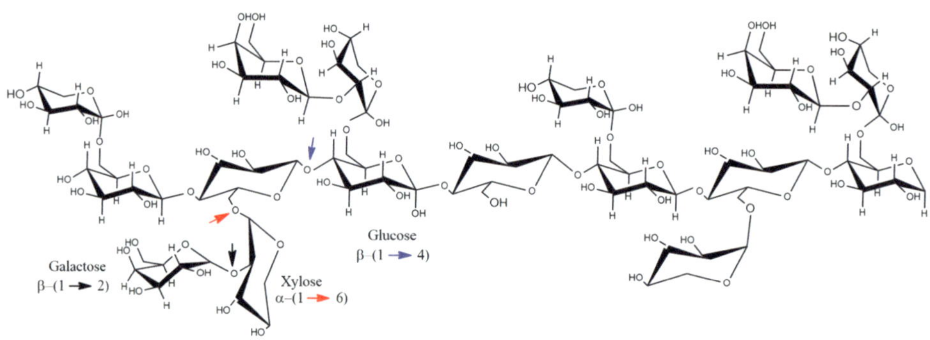

Figure 2.
Xyloglucan structure. As a hemicellulose, they have a backbone composed of β-(1,4)-linked glucans, and conversely to galactomannan structure, xyloglucans present β-(1,2)-linked galactosyl residues. This latter can also be found branched with an α-l-fucosyl residue. However, storage xyloglucan is not fucosylated.

3.2.2 Exudate gums (Arabic, tragacanth and cashew gum)

Exudate gums are hydrocolloids of high molecular weight and viscous appearance, derived from the exudates of branches and bark of the trunks of some plant species. In order to obtain these compounds, a process called gummosis must occur, phenomenon generated as a physiological defense response by chemical, physical and biological stimulus [28]. Chemically, they are made of a complex structure found in arabinogalactans, galacturonans, glucoronomannan or glucoronomannan of acid nature, branched and replaced by major elements (C, H, O and N), inorganic ions and secondary metabolites synthesized from the phenylpropanoid pathway (tannins, terpenoids and other phenolic compounds) [29].

Arabic gum (AG) is a polysaccharide with complex and branched structures (adhesive and cohesive properties) composed of side and main-chains with β(1,3) and (1,6), respectively, and D-galactopyranosyl, α-L-arabinofuranosyl, α-L-rhamnopyranosyl and β-D-glucopyran units. In some cases, GA is covalently associated with protein fractions and a high content of hydroxyproline, leucine, serine and proline residues [30]. Among its recognized pharmacological properties, we can cite its performance as mucous and intestinal anti-inflammatory, antibacterial and antioxidant, biochemical factors that are probably influential in the wound healing process [31–33].

Tragacanth gum (TG) is an anionic acid branched hetero-polymer with residual units of arabinose, glucose, xylose, galactose rhamnose, fucose and galacturonic acid [32], and TG has important biological characteristics, such as biodegradable and biocompatible biomaterials, resulting in suitable materials in the design of hybrid scaffolds with pharmaceutical applications, *development* of polymeric systems for *controlled release of drug* and guided tissue regeneration [34].

Similar to the polymer gums described above, cashew tree gum is extracted from *Anacardium* genus species, which are abundant Brazilian Northeast. The chemical structure is composed of a main-chain of β-galactose (1–3) and branched-bonds (1–6), containing side-residues of glucuronic acid, 4-O-methyl glucuronic arabinose, rhamnose, xylose, glucose and mannose [32]. The biochemical characteristics associated with biological activities demonstrate anti-inflammatory properties, regulators of oxidative stress and reactive oxygen species, antibacterial and gastroprotective effect [35].

3.3 Proteins

3.3.1 Latex proteases

Latex is produced and stored by laticifer ducts found in some plant species. This fluid is a rich source of natural compounds such as secondary metabolites, glycosides and proteases [36]. Latex proteins have been studied by several researchers as innovative natural compounds for biomedical applications [37]. Among the most common macromolecules from protein origin are cysteine and serine peptidases, also known as latex proteases or latex peptidases. These macromolecules provide the front line of defense against natural enemies in plants acting by synergism with others latex sap proteins [36].

Proteases are also present in animals and humans, and these enzymes have gained notoriety in medical and pharmaceutical field due to their proteolysis functions, specificity and bioactivity [38]. In human biological systems, proteases such as metalloproteinases are endogenously released by fibroblasts, macrophages, mast cells and endothelial cells after injury in extracellular matrix [39]. These enzymes initially participate in the inflammatory phase of healing by debriding the wound necrotic tissue and contributing to collagen remodeling and reduction of scar tensile strength, the later phase of cicatricial process [40]. Proteases and their inhibitors also contribute to degradation and deposition of ECM, creating a balance that is essential for the adequate and coordinated cutaneous wound healing [41].

The modulation of ECM proteases with laticifer proteins has been used as a strategy to improve the performance of healing processes in acute and chronic wounds [42]. Recent advances in plant latex biotechnology has contributed to study the pharmacological properties of proteases-rich fractions from *Calotropis procera* latex revealing its potential role in procoagulation and blood clot hydrolysis [43], modulation of inflammation [44, 45] and enhanced wound healing in animal models using biomembranes of polyvinyl alcohol as vehicle for releasing laticifer proteins [46, 47]. In addition, a phytomodulatory galactomannan-based hydrogel has been successfully used to carrier latex proteases from *C. procera* in experimental excisional wound models. It was observed a synergic effect between both galactomannan and proteases macromolecules, enhancing the healing [48].

3.3.2 Lectins

Lectins (from Latin "*legere,*" to pick out or choose) are proteins or glycoproteins found in nonimmune nature which can specifically recognize and reversibly bind carbohydrate moieties without altering the covalent structure of their glycosyl ligands. Indeed, this attractive characteristic distinguishes lectins from other carbohydrate binding proteins and enzymes. They are also widely distributed in the plant kingdom, usually from leguminous seed origin and play crucial roles and functions in biological processes such as molecular recognition, storage proteins and plant defense mechanisms. Their interaction with glycosyl ligands occurs mainly through hydrogen bonds, van der Waals' forces, hydrophobic interactions and, less frequently, electrostatic interactions [49]. Here, we emphasize lectins from jackfruit, breadfruit and chempedak (**Figure 3**) and their biological applications.

Lectins were first discovered in plants and, although ubiquitously distributed in nature (animals, insects, viruses, fungi and bacteria), and the majority have been characterized from plant protein extracts, reflecting ease of extraction and relatively high yields usually via a simple one-step affinity chromatographic method [50]. After the discovery of jacalin, novel lectins sharing high homology to it were placed into a family of jacalin-related lectins (JRL), now divided into two different subgroups. The first comprises galactose-specific lectins (gJRL) and a few other Moraceae lectins, which exhibit specificity toward galactose and are built up of subunits consisting of a short β chain and a long α chain. The second is the mannose-binding subgroup (mJRL), which occurs in different plant families with the lectins exhibiting exclusive specificity toward glucose/mannose residues with the binding subunits contained within a single polypeptide chain [51, 52].

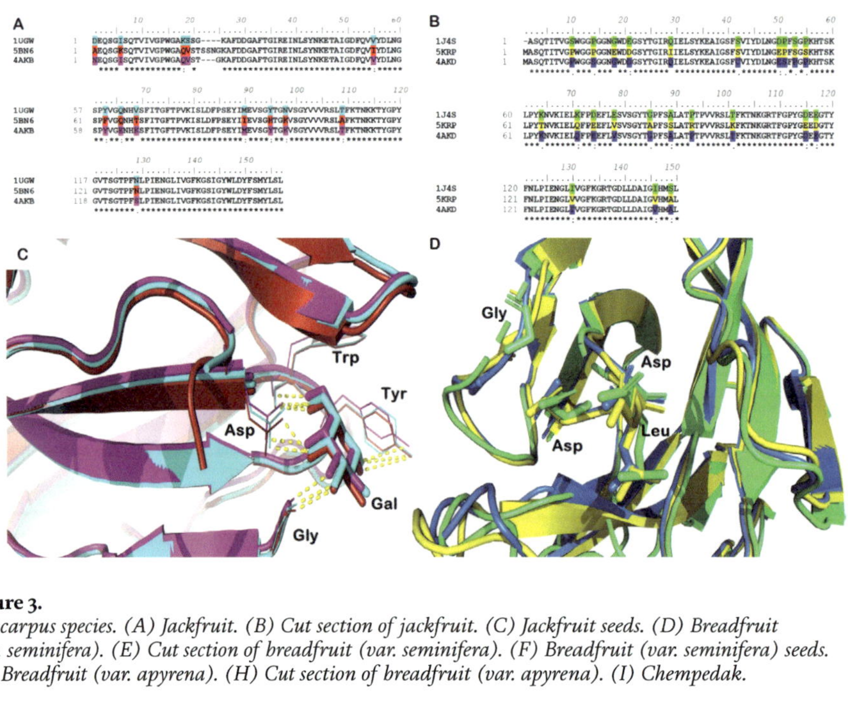

Figure 3.
Artocarpus species. (A) Jackfruit. (B) Cut section of jackfruit. (C) Jackfruit seeds. (D) Breadfruit (var. seminifera). (E) Cut section of breadfruit (var. seminifera). (F) Breadfruit (var. seminifera) seeds. (G) Breadfruit (var. apyrena). (H) Cut section of breadfruit (var. apyrena). (I) Chempedak.

3.3.2.1 Artocarpus lectins

Artocarpus is a genus comprising about 60 trees and shrubs of Southeast Asian and Pacific origin, belonging to the Moraceae family; all species are lactiferous with leaves, twigs, and stems producing milky sap. The name is derived from the Greek words *artos* ("bread") and *karpos* ("fruit"). Although most species of *Artocarpus* are restricted to Southeast Asia, such as *A. hypargyreus* (kwai muk), *A. lakoocha* (lakoocha), *A. kemando* (pudau), *A. hirsutus* (anjily), *A. chama* (chaplaish) and *A. odoratissimus* (marang), several species are widely distributed and cultivated throughout the tropics due to their edible fruits and timber. These include *A. heterophyllus* (jackfruit), *A. altilis* and *A. integer* (cempedak, also known as chempedak) [53–55], well-known species conspicuous as substantial sources of plant lectins which are readily recovered from their seed flour.

3.3.2.1.1 Jackfruit (jacalin, ArtinM and jackin)

The species has an extensive record of use in folk medicine including treatment of asthma, dermatitis, anemia, diarrhea and fever; antisyphilitic and anthelmintic properties; sedative effects in convulsions; and also wound healing properties [56]. Indeed, jackfruit are in high demand in areas such as cosmeceutical, pharmaceutical and natural food handling for supplement markets, due to numerous studies on phytochemical and pharmacological properties of all parts of the plant (pulp, leaf, root and bark) [57, 58].

Extracts and metabolites from jackfruit possess several useful bioactive compounds and may confer multiple health-promoting effects for heart and skin disorders and to treat ulcers and cancer [59]. Moreover, new studies of jackfruit properties provide additional biological findings consistent with antibacterial, antitubercular, antiviral, antifungal, antiplatelet and antiarthritic actions, thereby indicating therapeutic applications [56].

The occurrence of jacalin, the D-galactose-binding lectin from *A. integrifolia* seeds was first reported in 1979 [60] and found to exceed 50% of the protein in jackfruit crude seed extracts. This is also the case for galactose-binding lectins in the *Artocarpus* genus such as frutalin and CGB (chempedak galactose-binding). Jacalin is a tetrameric two-chain lectin of 65 kDa combining a heavy α-chain of 133 amino acids and light β-chain of 20–21 amino acid to form a 3D structure as a single globular unit. By SDS-PAGE, this lectin shows two bands between 20 and 14 kDa, which correspond to glycosylated and slightly or non-glycosylated forms, respectively [61].

The carbohydrate-binding site (CBS) of jacalin mainly involves residues Gly1, Tyr78, Val80, Gly121, Tyr122, Trp123 and Asp125. In D-galactose-jacalin complexes, the O4 hydroxyl group of the galactose axial position forms hydrogen bonds with the side chain of Asp125 and the terminal amino group of Gly1. If O4 is at the equatorial position, as in glucose and mannose, Asp125 can still interact with O4, but not the amino group. This explains the high specificity of jacalin for galactose compared to glucose and mannose at the primary binding site. Additionally, the post-translational cleavage and removal of the "T-S-S-N" peptide linker assure a stronger hydrogen bond connecting the α- and β-chains, as non-cleavage leaves a neutral peptide NH group [62, 63].

Further studies post-discovery of jacalin revealed that jackfruit seed extracts also possess small amounts of a D-mannose-binding lectin [64]. Previously named artocarpin, the term was provisionally replaced by the name KM+; the lectin had become confused with distinct substances from *Artocarpus* spp. which were similarly designated. Additionally, artocarpin was used to name the galactose-binding lectin in *Artocarpus lakoocha* seeds [65].

The origin of the name KM+ comes from the successive affinity chromatography steps in immobilized D-galactose matrices to remove jacalin (retained fraction J). The unretained fraction was called K, while M+ refers to the retained fraction on immobilized mannose matrices. Nevertheless, there remained confusion over this adopted nomenclature, which led to the proposal for a rational name change to ArtinM based on the universal code for plant proteins. This takes into account both a lectin's origin and specificity of sugar recognition [66]. Hereafter, we will apply ArtinM to include early work and mentions of KM+ (artocarpin).

ArtinM is a single polypeptide of 150 amino acids devoid of covalently attached carbohydrates with four isolectins and a pI range of 5–6.5, sharing 52% sequence identity with jacalin [67]. Unlike jacalin, there are no aromatic residues on the CBS of ArtinM, comprising Gly15, Asp138, Leu139 and Asp141. Indeed, it is believed that the galactose specificity of jacalin was achieved by a two-step process with ArtinM as its putative precursor: mutation of key aliphatic residues close to the sugar binding pocket to aromatic ones; and then cleavage of a short loop, a key step as it creates a positively charged N-terminal which interacts specifically with O4 at the axial position [68, 69].

Besides jacalin and ArtinM, jackfruit seeds are the source of a third lectin named jackin due to its affinity for chitin. Nevertheless, its low yield from natural sources still hampers further characterization, though this might soon be overcome with high-yield heterologous production in microbial systems [70].

3.3.2.1.2 Breadfruit

The Pacific Islands are the center of origin and diversity of breadfruit (*A. altilis*), sometimes referred to as *A. communis* or *A. incisa*. The species was derived from a seeded, diploid ancestor, *A. camansi,* giving two varieties, one seeded (var. seminifera) whose rind spines are as prominent as those on jackfruit, and one seedless (var. apyrena), which presents a spineless outer layer. The latter is well-appreciated by local Brazilians when cooked, because of its large starchy content of compound fruits with high levels of minerals and provitamin A carotenoids [53, 55, 71]. Breadfruit flour was approved in 2016 by the US Food and Drug Administration (FDA) as a food Generally Recognized as Safe (GRAS).

As of 1983, our group started to survey lectins in *A. incisa* seeds and found lectins with similar behavior to those in jackfruit seeds [72]. Breadfruit seeds are composed of a high-water content (up to 60%) and moderate protein content (12.25% of dry weight). Most of this protein is recovered as frutalin in chromatographic methods using crude extracts of seed flour. Therefore, frutalin is the most abundant lectin of this species, presenting multiple-binding properties in which the same CBS recognizes a range of different ligands, although it has higher affinities for α-D-galactose monosaccharides and complex carbohydrates that contain Galα1–3 glycans [73].

The CBS of frutalin in the binding of galactose is dominated by hydrogen bonding through O1, O3, O5 and O6 and backbone/side chain hydroxyl groups. Similar to the Moraceae lectins, the CBS of frutalin is located in a domain close to the N-terminus of the α chain, consisting of four key residues Gly25, Tyr146, Trp147 and Asp149. About 10 interactions occur, involving the C1 hydroxyl to residue Tyr146, hydroxyl C3 to residue Gly25, hydroxyl C4 to residues Gly25 and Asp149, and hydroxyl C6 to residues Tyr146, Trp147 and Asp149 [74]. Moreover, there is evidence to suggest that frutalin possesses stereospecificity, capable of specifically binding α-D-galactose, since it was previously isolated on a cross-linked galactomannan column, but not on β-galactosyl-immobilized matrices [73, 75].

Frutapin (FTP) is the next most abundant lectin in breadfruit seed extracts. Preliminary, FTP investigations began in 1998, describing three different lectins with distinct carbohydrate recognition within the same species [76]. However, further studies proved difficult since native FTP was hampered by very low yields and contamination with Frutalin, a notable factor as frutalin binds diverse sugar moieties and has high abundance in plant extracts. Recombinant FTP production is now a feasible approach to circumvent this problem, allowing large-scale heterologous expression to give continuous supplies for further characterization and to improve potency, particularly for biomedical applications [77].

FTP is a hololectin defined as a homotetramer with an identical CBS per protomer, able to bind either the same or structurally similar sugars. The CBS is formed of four residues, namely Gly16, Asp139, Leu140 and Asp142, distributed in a few loops connecting the strands β5 and β6, β7 and β8, and β11 and β12. Several hydrogen bonds (HB) occur in FTP-glucose and FTP-mannose complexes involving Gly16, Leu90, Gly138, Asp139, Leu140, Asp142 and O3, O4, O5, O6 of the carbohydrates. In MD simulations, Lys60 plays an important role forming salt bridges with Asp139 in FTP-glucose complexes, reducing the interaction between this former residue and mannose and minimizing the repulsion of the mannose hydroxyl groups with oxygen. In this case, mannose was more completely surrounded in the carbohydrate-binding site and also stabilized by indirect interaction with Asp139 through water molecules. This local structuring is more stable in the case of mannose than glucose, indicating a higher affinity of FTP for mannose residues than glucose [78].

Further studies of breadfruit seeds also revealed a lectin similar to jackin, named frutackin. Both lectins have a 14 kDa polypeptide chain, built up of three chains linked by disulfide bonds, the partial amino acid sequences of the two lectins showing their homology to each other in terms of molecular mass, secondary structure, and primary sequence, but not to other plant chitin-binding proteins. Both jackin and frutackin inhibit the growth of *F. moniliforme* and *S. cerevisiae* [70].

3.3.2.1.3 Chempedak

Although widely known in the tropics as chempedak or chempedak, *Artocarpus integer* (Thumb.) Merr. is native to India with similar fruits to jackfruit. The *A. integer* species is rich in phenolic compounds, presenting a strong cytotoxic activity against murine leukemia P-388 [79]. Moreover, a chempedak paste of the inner bark prevents infection and helps healing when applied on wounds, as well as heated leaf extract [80].

Chempedak galactose-binding lectin (CGB) is found in high levels *A. integer* seed flour extracts. The lectin's bioactivity was first noted when extracts were tested for selective stimulation of peripheral blood mononuclear cells; at 20 μg/mL CGB stimulated proliferation of T-lymphocyte populations [81, 82]. Like frutalin and jacalin, CGB is transcribed as a propeptide and then post-translationally processed into a typical gJRL lectin, having a 13-kDa α-chain (133 amino acids) and a 2.1-kDa β-chain (21 amino acids). CGB has six different amino-acids compared to jacalin, giving 97% identity for their amino-acid sequences [83].

As with jacalin complexes, the interactions are well conserved, presenting the same CBS. In Gal-CGB complexes, the O atoms on the sugar ring are bound with the side-chain and main-chain N and O atoms on the α chain (O3 and Gly1 N; O4 and Gly1 N and Asp125 OD1; O6 and Trp123 O, Trp123 N and Tyr122 N; and O5 and Tyr122 N). Similarly, GalNac-CGB complexes present bound disaccharide in the same region though hydrogen bonds (O3 and Gly1 N; O4 and Gly1 N and Asp125 OD1; and O6 and Asp125 OD1). Also, there are a number of hydrophobic interactions contributed by Tyr78, Gly121 and Tyr122. Although closely related to jacalin's structure, CGB was unable to bind mannose as judged by isothermal calorimetry and co-crystallization studies. It is believed that this change in CGB specificity is caused by subtle differences in the environment near the sugar-binding site, including solvent molecules.

Extracts of *Artocarpus integer* seeds are a source of CMB, previously termed chempedak lectin-M [84]. The lectin is ~20-fold more abundant than ArtinM in crude extracts of *A. heterophyllus* seeds. Structural studies reveal CMB to be a 64-kDa tetramer with some of the polypeptides being disulfide-linked to give dimers. The functional activity of CMB was assessed by studying interactions with different isotypes of human immunoglobulins: strong binding to IgE and IgM was noted, unlike CGB and jacalin which strongly interact with IgA1. The lectin also shows a similar pattern of carbohydrate binding specificity to ArtinM with Man-α-1–3Man the most potent inhibitor, followed by methyl-α-D-mannopyranose and D-mannose [84].

It appears that the *Artocarpus* genus employs a plurality of lectins, though to date few of these lectins have been purified and functionally characterized. Nevertheless, a consistent pattern is that *Artocarpus* seeds contain more than one lectin with distinct carbohydrate recognition features [70, 76]. Altogether, the JRL family is complex with a vast diversity in biochemical properties and activities, which have drawn much attention because of their pivotal biomedical applications. Owing to carbohydrate-binding interactions of plant lectins with cell wall glycoproteins, they are promising targets to selectively modulate immune responses in plants. Hence, it is important to delineate the molecular details of lectin binding to CBS domains and how downstream activation of cellular immune signaling proceeds [85]. In this context, it is of particular note that *Artocarpus* lectins have a distinct repertoire of biological activities, despite their high sequence and structural homology, as can be seen in **Figure 4**.

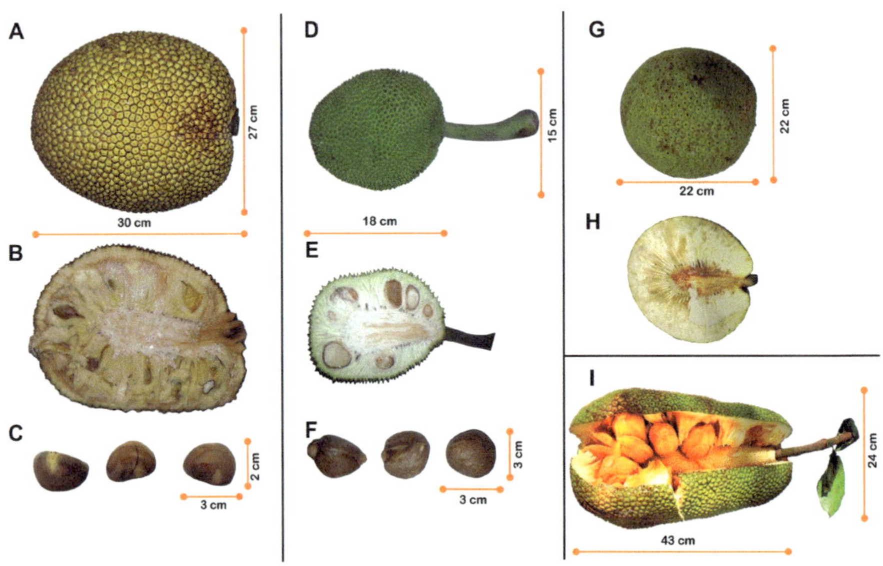

Figure 4.
Sequence alignment using Clustal W and structural superposition of Artocarpus *lectins. (A) Sequence alignment of galactose-binding lectins: Jacalin (PDB 1UGW), Frutalin (PDB 5BN6), and CGB (PDB 4AKB). (B) Sequence alignment of mannose-binding lectins: ArtinM (PDB 1J4S), frutapin (PDB 5KRP) and CMB (PDB 4AKD). (C) Structural superposition of galactose-binding lectins with their carbohydrate interacting residues in complex with D-galactose: jacalin (cyan), frutalin (red) and CGB (magenta). (D) Structural superposition of mannose-binding lectins with the carbohydrate interacting residues highlighted: ArtinM (green), frutapin (yellow) and CMB (blue).*

4. Recent advances using plant biomaterials for wound healing

The worldwide increasing number of chronic-wound patients has driven an intense effort in the wound-care market in search of low cost and effective wound healing technologies [86]. Therefore, much of this knowledge is eligible for patents that play an important role in identifying technology development trends [86].

In the following table, we highlight the main efforts in the last 5 years on the development of biomaterials using plant macromolecules as source of biomolecules with potential for wound healing applications (**Table 1**).

Title	Plant biomaterial	Description	IPC code	Ref.
Necrotic tissue composition remover for wound healing	Protease mixture	An aqueous gel is carrier for a protease mixture for removing necrotic tissue in chronic wounds.	A61K38/4873	[87]
Compound preparation for wound healing and postpartum rehabilitation	Hydrolysate: synthases I, alkaline protease and papain	Compound preparations that promote blood circulation and wound healing.	A61K 36/00	[88]
Dead Sea Water and apple of Sodom extract compositions and uses thereof	*C. procera*	The compositions may be used for topical administration in wound healing.	—	[89]
Therapeutic composition for wound healing	β-glucan and at least one secondary polysaccharide group consisting of arabinogalactan, fucoidan, pectin and galactomannan	Therapeutic composition as a potent stimulator for wound healing.	A61K 31/716	[90]
Anti-adhesion material with antibacterial and healing properties	Xyloglucan	The material is used for preventing reoccurrence of adhesion after adhesion loss operation, and meanwhile has functions of preventing bacteria and promoting wound healing.	A61L31/041	[91]
Plant hemicelluloses and lectins formulations with healing activity	Hemicelluloses and plant lectins	Hydrogels and biomembranes are used to treat wounds, abrasions, burns, varicose ulcers, decubitus ulcers, open superficial wounds with or without infection.	A61K 31/736	[92]

IPC: International Patent Classification.

Table 1.
Recent patents of plant biomaterials for wound healing.

5. Conclusion

As an orchestrated sequence of biochemical and cellular events for tissue repair, the healing process becomes a challenging in a way to develop a universal dressing, attending all the sorts of wound and lesions. It is here that biomaterials are notably relevant for biomedical applications once multiple properties of them can be combined in formulations of new treatments strategies of wound healing and repair. Many plants have been used traditionally in therapeutic treatments of lesions, which make them a remarkable source of biomolecules to wound-care market.

Author details

Felipe Domingos de Sousa[1]*, Francisco Rogênio da Silva Mendes[2], Jose Jovanny Bermudez-Sierra[2], Ayrles Fernanda Brandão da Silva[3], Mirele da Silveira Vasconcelos[4], Tamiris de Fátima Goebel de Souza[5], Marília de Oliveira Nunes[5], Antônio Eufrásio Vieira-Neto[2], Marcos Roberto Lourenzoni[6], Rosueti Diógenes de Oliveira-Filho[7], Adriana Rolim Campos[2], Renato de Azevedo Moreira[2] and Ana Cristina de Oliveira Monteiro-Moreira[2]

1 Department of Physics, Federal University of Ceará, Fortaleza, Ceará, Brazil

2 Northeast Biotechnology Network (RENORBIO), Centre of Experimental Biology (Nubex), University of Fortaleza (UNIFOR), Fortaleza, Ceará, Brazil

3 Department of Biochemistry and Molecular Biology, Federal University of Ceará (UFC), Fortaleza, Ceará, Brazil

4 Federal Institute of Education, Science and Technology of Ceará, Baturité, Ceará, Brazil

5 Department of Physiology and Pharmacology, Drug Research and Development Center (NPDM), Federal University of Ceara, Fortaleza, Ceará, Brazil

6 Fiocruz, Fundação Oswaldo Cruz—Ceará, Drugs and Biopharmaceuticals Development Group: Evolution, in silico and in vitro of Biomolecules, Fortaleza, Ceará, Brazil

7 Department of Clinical and Toxicological Analysis, Federal University of Ceará, Fortaleza, Ceará, Brazil

*Address all correspondence to: fdsousa@yahoo.com.br

References

[1] Sorg H, Tilkorn DJ, Hager S, Hauser J, Mirastschijski U. Skin wound healing: An update on the current knowledge and concepts. European Surgical Research. 2017;**58**(1-2):81-94

[2] Kathju S, Gallo PH, Satish L. Scarless integumentary wound healing in the mammalian fetus: Molecular basis and therapeutic implications. Birth Defects Research. Part C, Embryo Today: Reviews. 2012;**96**(3):223-236

[3] Han G, Ceilley R. Chronic wound healing: A review of current management and treatments. Advances in Therapy. 2017;**34**(3):599-610

[4] Chaudhari AA, Vig K, Baganizi DR, Sahu R, Dixit S, Dennis V, et al. Future prospects for scaffolding methods and biomaterials in skin tissue engineering: A review. The International Journal of Molecular Sciences. 2016;**17**(12):1-31

[5] Nicholas MN, Jeschke MG, Amini-Nik S. Methodologies in creating skin substitutes. Cellular and Molecular Life Sciences. 2016;**73**(18):3453-3472

[6] Das S, Baker AB. Biomaterials and nanotherapeutics for enhancing skin wound healing. Frontiers in Bioengineering and Biotechnology. 2016;**4**(82):1-20

[7] Gonzalez AC, Costa TF, Andrade ZD, Medrado AR. Wound healing—A literature review. Anais Brasileiros de Dermatologia. 2016;**91**(5):614-620

[8] Golebiewska EM, Poole AW. Platelet secretion: From haemostasis to wound healing and beyond. Blood Reviews. 2015;**29**(3):153-162

[9] Zhao R, Liang H, Clarke E, Jackson C, Xue M. Inflammation in chronic wounds. International Journal of Molecular Sciences. 2016;**17**(12):1-14

[10] Martin P, Nunan R. Cellular and molecular mechanisms of repair in acute and chronic wound healing. The British Journal of Dermatology. 2015;**173**(2):370-378

[11] Hesketh M, Sahin KB, West ZE, Murray RZ. Macrophage phenotypes regulate scar formation and chronic wound healing. International Journal of Molecular Sciences. 2017;**18**(7):1-10

[12] Darby IA, Laverdet B, Bonté F, Desmoulière A. Fibroblasts and myofibroblasts in wound healing. Clinical, Cosmetic and Investigational Dermatology. 2014;**7**:301-311

[13] Georgescu M, Marinas O, Popa M, Stan T, Lazar V, Bertesteanu SV, et al. Natural compounds for wound healing. In: da Fonseca CJV, editor. Worldwide Wound Healing—Innovation in Natural and Conventional Methods. Portugal: IntechOpen; 2016. pp. 61-89

[14] Pérez-Recalde M, Ruiz Arias IE, Hermida ÉB. Could essential oils enhance biopolymers performance for wound healing? A systematic review. Phytomedicine. 2018;**38**:57-65

[15] Bassolé IHN, Juliani HR. Essential oils in combination and their antimicrobial properties. Molecules. 2012;**17**(4):3989-4006

[16] Raut JS, Karuppayil SM. A status review on the medicinal properties of essential oils. Industrial Crops and Products. 2014;**62**:250-264

[17] Pesavento G, Calonico C, Bilia AR, Barnabei M, Calesini F, Addona R, et al. Antibacterial activity of oregano, Rosmarinus and thymus essential oils against *Staphylococcus aureus* and listeria monocytogenes in beef meatballs. Food Control. 2015;**54**:188-199

[18] Guimarães AG, Quintans JSS, Quintans-Júnior LJ. Monoterpenes with analgesic activity—A systematic review. Phytotherapy Research. 2013;**27**(1):1-15

[19] Dyer GA. A primer on seed and nut biology, improvement, and use. In: Preedy VR, Watson RR, Patel VB, editors. Nuts and Seeds in Health and Disease Prevention. New York: Elsevier Inc.; 2011. pp. 5-13

[20] Pauly M, Gille S, Liu L, Mansoori N, de Souza A, Schultink A, et al. Hemicellulose biosynthesis. Planta. 2013;**238**:627

[21] Scheller HV, Ulvskov P. Hemicelluloses. Annual Review of Plant Biology. 2010;**61**(1):263-289

[22] Buckeridge MS. Seed cell wall storage polysaccharides: Models to understand cell wall biosynthesis and degradation. Plant Physiology. 2010;**154**(3):1017-1023

[23] Bento JF, Mazzaro I, De Almeida Silva LM, De Azevedo MR, Ferreira MLC, Reicher F, et al. Diverse patterns of cell wall mannan/galactomannan occurrence in seeds of the Leguminosae. Carbohydrate Polymers. 2013;**92**(1):192-199

[24] Prajapati VD, Jani GK, Moradiya NG, Randeria NP, Nagar BJ, Naikwadi NN, et al. Galactomannan: A versatile biodegradable seed polysaccharide. The International Journal of Biological Macromolecules. 2013;**60**:83-92

[25] Srivastava M, Kapoor VP. Seed galactomannans: An overview. Chemistry and Biodiversity. 2005;**2**:295-317

[26] Cosgrove DJ. Expansive growth of plant cell walls. Plant Physiology and Biochemistry. 2000;**38**(1-2):109-124

[27] Picone P, Antonietta M, Ajovalasit A, Giacomazza D, Dispenza C, Di M. Biocompatibility , hemocompatibility and antimicrobial properties of xyloglucan-based hydrogel fi lm for wound healing application. International Journal of Biological Macromolecules. 2019;**121**:784-795

[28] Rana V, Rai P, Tiwary AK, Singh RS, Kennedy JF, Knill CJ. Modified gums: Approaches and applications in drug delivery. Carbohydrate Polymers. 2011;**83**(3):1031-1047

[29] Shen T, Yuan H-Q, Wan W-Z, Wang X-L. Cycloartane-type triterpenoids from the resinous exudates of *Commiphora opobalsamum*. Journal of Natural Products. 2008;**71**(1):81-86

[30] Musa HH, Ahmed AA, Musa TH. Chemistry, biological, and pharmacological properties of gum Arabic. In: Mérillon JM, Ramawat KG, editors. Bioactive Molecules in Food, 2019. Switzerland: Springer; 2019. pp. 797-814

[31] Ali BH, Ziada A, Blunden G. Biological effects of gum arabic: A review of some recent research. Food and Chemical Toxicology. 2009;**47**(1):1-8

[32] Nussinovitch A. Plant Gum Exudates of the World. Sources, Distribution, Properties, and Applications. 1st ed. Boca Raton USA: CRC Press/Taylor & Francis; 2009. 430 p

[33] Zhang X, Liu W, Kang X, Wang Z, Bai J, Ji L. Stimulation of wound healing using bioinspired hydrogels with basic fibroblast growth factor (bFGF). International Journal of Nanomedicine. 2018;**13**:3897-3906

[34] Nazarzadeh Zare E, Makvandi P, Tay FR. Recent progress in the industrial and biomedical applications of tragacanth gum: A review. Carbohydrate Polymers. 2019;**212**:450-467

[35] Moreira BR, Batista KA, Castro EG, Lima EM, Fernandes KF. A

bioactive film based on cashew gum polysaccharide for wound dressing applications. Carbohydrate Polymers. 2015;**122**:69-76

[36] Ramos MV, Demarco D, da Costa Souza IC, de Freitas CDT. Laticifers, latex, and their role in plant defense. Trends in Plant Science. 2019;**24**(6):553-567

[37] Ujwala K, Karpagam N. Potential therapeutical values of plant latices. International Journal of Medicinal and Aromatic Plants. 2013;**3**(2):317-325

[38] Gurumallesh P, Alagu K, Ramakrishnan B, Muthusamy S. A systematic reconsideration on proteases. The International Journal of Biological Macromolecules. 2019;**128**:254-267

[39] Reiss MJ, Han YP, Garcia E, Goldberg M, Yu H, Garner WL. Matrix metalloproteinase-9 delays wound healing in a murine wound model. Surgery. 2010;**147**(2):295-302

[40] Younan GJ, Heit YI, Dastouri P, Kekhia H, Xing W, Gurish MF, et al. Mast cells are required in the proliferation and remodeling phases of microdeformational wound therapy. Plastic and Reconstructive Surgery. 2011;**128**(6):649-658

[41] McCarty SM, Percival SL. Proteases and delayed wound healing. Advances in Wound Care. 2013;**2**(8):438-447

[42] Westby Maggie J, Dumville Jo C, Stubbs N, Norman G, Cullum N, Westby MJ, et al. Protease-modulating matrix treatments for healing venous leg ulcers. The Cochrane Database of Systematic Reviews. 2016;**2015**(12):1-18

[43] Ramos MV, Viana CA, Silva AFB, Freitas CDT, Figueiredo IST, Oliveira RSB, et al. Proteins derived from latex of *C. procera* maintain coagulation homeostasis in septic mice and exhibit thrombin- and plasmin-like activities. Naunyn-Schmiedeberg's Archives of Pharmacology. 2012;**385**(5):455-463

[44] Freitas APF, Bitencourt FS, Brito GAC, De Alencar NMN, Ribeiro RA, Lima RCP, et al. Protein fraction of *Calotropis procera* latex protects against 5-fluorouracil-induced oral mucositis associated with downregulation of pivotal pro-inflammatory mediators. Naunyn-Schmiedeberg's Archives of Pharmacology. 2012;**385**(10):981-990

[45] Ramos MV, Oliveira JS, Figueiredo JG, Figueiredo IST, Kumar VL, Bitencourt FS, et al. Involvement of NO in the inhibitory effect of *Calotropis procera* latex protein fractions on leukocyte rolling, adhesion and infiltration in rat peritonitis model. Journal of Ethnopharmacology. 2009;**125**(3):387-392

[46] De Figueiredo IST, Ramos MV, Ricardo NMPS, Gonzaga MLDC, Pinheiro RSP, De Alencar NMN. Efficacy of a membrane composed of polyvinyl alcohol as a vehicle for releasing of wound healing proteins belonging to latex of *Calotropis procera*. Process Biochemistry. 2014;**49**(3):512-519

[47] Ramos MV, de Alencar NMN, de Oliveira RSB, Freitas LBN, Aragão KS, de Andrade TAM, et al. Wound healing modulation by a latex protein-containing polyvinyl alcohol biomembrane. Naunyn-Schmiedeberg's Archives of Pharmacology. 2016;**389**(7):747-756

[48] Vasconcelos MS, Souza TFG, Figueiredo IS, Sousa ET, Sousa FD, Moreira RA, et al. A phytomodulatory hydrogel with enhanced healing effects. Phytotherapy Research. 2018:1-10

[49] Peumans WJ, Van Damme EJ. Lectins as plant defense proteins. Plant Physiology. 1995;**109**(2):347-352

[50] Dang L, Van Damme EJM. Toxic proteins in plants. Phytochemistry. 2015;**117**(1):51-64

[51] Bourne Y, Zamboni V, Barre A, Peumans WJ, Van Damme EJM, Rougé P. Helianthus tuberosus lectin reveals a widespread scaffold for mannose- binding lectins. Structure. 1999;**7**(12):1473-1482

[52] Wright CS. New folds of plant lectins. Current Opinion in Structural Biology. 1997;**7**(5):631-636

[53] Zerega NJC, Ragone D, Motley TJ. Systematics and species limits of breadfruit. Systematic Botany. 2005;**30**(3):603-615

[54] de Lopes MMA, de Souza KO, de Silva EO. Cempedak—*Artocarpus champeden*. In: Rodrigues S, de Silva EO, de Brito ES, editors. Exotic Fruits Reference Guide. London: Wolff, Andre Gerhard; 2018. pp. 121-126

[55] Ragone D. Breadfruit—*Artocarpus altilis* (Parkinson) Fosberg. In: Rodrigues S, de Silva EO, de Brito ES, editors. Exotic Fruits Reference Guide. London: Wolff, Andre Gerhard; 2018. pp. 53-59

[56] Jagtap UB, Bapat VA. Artocarpus: A review of its traditional uses, phytochemistry and pharmacology. Journal of Ethnopharmacology. 2010;**129**:142-146

[57] Govindaraj D, Rajan M, Hatamleh AA, Munusamy MA. From waste to high-value product: Jackfruit peel derived pectin/apatite bionanocomposites for bone healing applications. The International Journal of Biological Macromolecules. 2018;**106**:293-301

[58] Zhu H, Zhang Y, Tian J, Chu Z. Effect of a new shell material—Jackfruit seed starch on novel flavor microcapsules containing vanilla oil. Industrial Crops and Products. 2018;**112**:47-52

[59] Swami SB, Thakor NJ, Haldankar PM, Kalse SB. Jackfruit and its many functional components as related to human health: A review. Comprehensive Reviews in Food Science and Food Safety. 2012;**11**(6):565-576

[60] Chatterjee B, Vaith P, Chatterjee S, Karduck D, Uhlenbruck G. Comparative studies of new marker lectins for alkali-labile and alkali-stable carbohydrate chains in glycoproteins. The International Journal of Biochemistry. 1979;**10**(4):321-327

[61] Moreira RA, Ainouz IL. Lectins from seeds of jack fuit (*Artocarpus integrifolia L.*): Isolation and purification of two isolectins from the albumin fraction. Biologia Plantarum. 1981;**23**(3):186-192

[62] Sankaranarayanan R, Sekar K, Banerjee R, Sharma V, Surolia A, Vijayan M. A novel mode of carbohydrate recognition in jacalin, a Moraceae plant lectin with a β-prism fold. Nature Structural Biology. 1996;**3**(7):596-603

[63] Abhinav KV, Sharma K, Surolia A, Vijayan M. Distortion of the ligand molecule as a strategy for modulating binding affinity: Further studies involving complexes of jacalin with β-substituted disaccharides. IUBMB Life. 2017;**69**(2):72-78

[64] de Miranda-Santos IK, Mengel JO Jr, Bunn-Moreno MM, Campos-Neto A. Activation of T and B cells by a crude extract of *Artocarpus integrifolia* is mediated by a lectin distinct from jacalin. Journal of Immunological Methods. 1991;**140**(2):197-203

[65] Chowdhury S, Ahmed H, Chatterjee BP. Chemical modification studies of *Artocarpus lakoocha*

lectin artocarpin. Biochimie. 1991;**73**(5):563-571

[66] Pereira-da-Silva G, Roque-Barreira MC, Van Damme EJM. Artin M: A rational substitution for the names artocarpin and KM+. Immunology Letters. 2008;**119**(1-2):114-115

[67] DaSilva LLP, de Molfetta-Machado JB, Panunto-Castelo A, Denecke J, Goldman GH, Roque-Barreira MC, et al. cDNA cloning and functional expression of KM+, the mannose-binding lectin from *Artocarpus integrifolia* seeds. Biochimica et Biophysica Acta, General Subjects. 2005;**1726**(3):251-260

[68] Pratap JV, Jeyaprakash AA, Rani PG, Sekar K, Surolia A, Vijayan M. Crystal structures of artocarpin, a Moraceae lectin with mannose specificity, and its complex with methyl-alpha-D-mannose: Implications to the generation of carbohydrate specificity. The Journal of Molecular Biology. 2002;**317**(2):237-247

[69] Jeyaprakash AA, Srivastav A, Surolia A, Vijayan M. Structural basis for the carbohydrate specificities of artocarpin: Variation in the length of a loop as a strategy for generating ligand specificity. Journal of Molecular Biology. 2004;**338**(4):757-770

[70] Trindade MB, Lopes JLS, Soares-Costa A, Monteiro-Moreira AC, Moreira RA, Oliva MLV, et al. Structural characterization of novel chitin-binding lectins from the genus Artocarpus and their antifungal activity. Biochimica et Biophysica Acta, Proteins and Proteomics. 2006;**1764**(1):146-152

[71] Zerega N, Wiesner-Hanks T, Ragone D, Irish B, Scheffler B, Simpson S, et al. Diversity in the breadfruit complex (Artocarpus, Moraceae): Genetic characterization of critical germplasm. Tree Genetics and Genomes. 2015;**11**(1):1-26

[72] de Moreira RA, de Oliveira JTA. Lectins from the genus Artocarpus. Biologia Plantarum. 1983;**25**(5):343-348

[73] de Moreira RA, Castelo-Branco CC, de Monteiro ACO, Tavares RO, Beltramini LM. Isolation and partial characterization of a lectin from *Artocarpus incisa L*. seeds. Phytochemistry. 1998;**47**(7):1183-1188

[74] Vieira-neto AE. Caracterização estrutural da frutalina, uma lectina α-D-galactose ligante de sementes de artocarpus incisa e análise das suas bases moleculares de ligação à D-galactose [PhD Thesis]. Universidade Federal do Ceará; 2015

[75] De-Simone SG, Netto CC, Silva FP. Simple affinity chromatographic procedure to purify β-galactoside binding lectins. Journal of Chromatography, B: Analytical Technologies in the Biomedical and Life Sciences. 2006;**838**(2):135-138

[76] Monteiro-Moreira ACO. Caracterização estrutural de três lectinas apresentando especificidades por açúcar distintas, isoladas de sementes de fruta-pão (*Artocarpus incisa* L.) [PhD thesis]. Federal University of Ceará—UFC; 2002

[77] Oliveira C, Teixeira JA, Domingues L. Recombinant production of plant lectins in microbial systems for biomedical application—The frutalin case study. Frontiers in Plant Science. 2014;**5**:390

[78] de Sousa FD, da Silva BB, Furtado GP, de Carneiro IS, MDP L, Guan Y, et al. Frutapin, a lectin from *Artocarpus incisa* (breadfruit): Cloning, expression and molecular insights. Bioscience Reports. 2017;**37**(4):BSR20170969

[79] Syah YM, Juliawaty LD, Achmad SA, Hakim EH, Ghisalberti EL. Cytotoxic prenylated flavones from Artocarpus

champeden. Journal of Natural Medicines. 2006;**60**(4):308-312

[80] Farooq U, Malviya R, Sharma PK. Extraction and characterization of Artocarpus integer gum as pharmaceutical excipient. Polimery w Medycynie. 2014;**44**(2):69-74

[81] Hashim O, Gende G, Jaafar M. Lectin extracts of champedak seeds demonstrate selective stimulation of T lymphocyte proliferation. Biochemistry International. 1992;**27**(1):139-143

[82] Hashim OH, Ng CL, Gendeh GS, Jaafar MIN. Iga binding lectins isolated from distinct artocarpus species demonstrate differential specificity. Molecular Immunology. 1991;**28**(4-5):393-398

[83] Gabrielsen M, Abdul-Rahman PS, Othman S, Hashim OH, Cogdell RJ. Structures and binding specificity of galactose- and mannose-binding lectins from chempedak: Differences from jackfruit lectins. Acta Crystallographica Section F: Structural Biology Communications. 2014;**70**(6):709-716

[84] Lim SB, Chua CT, Hashim OH. Isolation of a mannose-binding and IgE- and IgM-reactive lectin from the seeds of Artocarpus integer. Journal of Immunological Methods. 1997;**209**(2):177-186

[85] Van Holle S, Van Damme EJM. Signaling through plant lectins: Modulation of plant immunity and beyond. Biochemical Society Transactions. 2018;**36**(2):221-247

[86] Gwak JH, Sohn SY. Identifying the trends in wound-healing patents for successful investment strategies. PLoS One. 2017;**12**(3):1-19

[87] Askurai E, Geblin D, Clayman M FD. Necrotic tissue composition remover for wound healing. Korea; 2018. KR20180104138A

[88] Maojun Y, Wang X, Dayuan Z GS. Compound preparation capable of promoting wound healing and postpartum rehabilitation. China; 2016. CN105770849A

[89] Cohen MP, Maor Z, Ish-Shalom E CD. Dead Sea Water and apple of Sodom extract compositions and uses thereof. 2017. WO2019130301A1

[90] Phipps W. Therapeutic composition for wound healing. United States; 2016. US20160256480A1

[91] Fanglian Y, Ershuai Z, Hong S. Anti-adhesion material with antibacterial and healing properties. China; 2016. CN106362221A

[92] de Sousa FD, de Moreira RA, Monteiro-Moreira ACO, Campos AR, Vasconselos PD. Plant hemicelluloses and lectins formulations with healing activity. Brazil; 2017. BR102017006983A2

Chapter 4

Modulation of Inflammatory Dynamics by Insulin to Promote Wound Recovery of Diabetic Ulcers

Pawandeep Kaur and Diptiman Choudhury

Abstract

About 5% of the world population is diabetic and are at a risk of slow non-recoverable wound formation. Estimated 15–25% of diabetic patients develop foot ulcers, 6% among them needing clinical attention among which 15–20% will need an amputation. This counts for around 50% of all traumatic amputation. Wound leads to activation of dynamic inflammatory cascade responsible for the healing process. But in diabetes, a persistent rise of pro-inflammatory cytokines and low anti-inflammatory cytokines blocks the dynamic cascade. Wounding induces various pro-inflammatory cytokines such as IL-1, IL-6, IL-12, IL-18, IFN-γ, and TNFs causing accumulation of free radicals leading to inflammation which become persistent in diabetes. Inhibition of proinflammatory cytokines drives the equilibrium towards the expression of anti-inflammatory cytokines such as IL4, IL-10, IL-11, IL-13, IFN-α, and TGF-β, which is necessary for the wound recovery process. Here in this chapter, the inflammatory modulatory roles of different drugs/formulations have been discussed to unravel their significance to promote wound recovery.

Keywords: diabetic wound, tissue inflammation, pro-inflammatory cytokines, anti-inflammatory cytokines, nanoformulation for wound recovery

1. Introduction

Over the last 25 years, there has been found a four-fold increase in the number of diabetes mellitus cases commonly called diabetes [1]. 422 million people worldwide in 2016 have been reported to have diabetes mellitus. Diabetes in the year 2012 was a cause of 1.5 million deaths worldwide; according to WHO (World Health Organization), diabetes becomes the 8th leading cause of death [2]. Diabetes mellitus is mainly identified by the presence free glucose at high or the chronic level in the body fluids like sweat, urine, blood, etc. [3]. The major reason for diabetes mellitus among others was the hormone-mediated metabolism regulation failure. Hormones like glucagon and insulin play an important role in regulating the level of blood sugar or maintaining its balance [4]. The sugar balance in blood is important for perfect functioning of human body [5]. High/chronic level of glucose in body fluids is responsible for different pathological conditions like infection susceptibility, leading to various diseases such as arthritis, hypertension, cardiovascular problems, cataract, retinopathy, neuropathy, damage of kidneys, damaging of blood vesicles, wound healing delay, etc. (**Figure 1**) [5, 6]. Due to the linkage of diabetes mellitus with other different diseases, the International Diabetes Foundation (IDF), in 2014, recorded that the 4.9 million lives loss and ~1.25% dead were diabetic patients, either directly by diabetes mellitus or indirectly through other diseases [7]. All these diseases are linked causing various effects on different body organs with various pathways; pathological/hyperglycemic conditions are linked with the inflammation of tissue [8]. Diabetes is responsible for lower gradation inflammation in a systemic way and leads to the promotion of different diseases like arthritis, retinopathy, etc. [9, 10].

One of the major problems associated with diabetes mellitus is inflammation in wounds and results in wound recovery delay [11]. The chronic wounds in diabetes mainly show the persistent increase in the level of pro-inflammatory cytokine and the absence of the signals, which are responsible for signals in the damaged tissues [12]. The treatments used in diabetes mellitus are also helpful in controlling the level of glucose blood and helps in delaying the further progression of other diseases linked with diabetes mellitus, like retinopathy, contract, arthritis, neuropathy, retinopathy, etc., but very less is known in the literature about diabetes mellitus treatment's effects on diabetic wound recovery [13]. Wound results in release of the pro-inflammatory cytokines such as interleukin-6 (IL-6), IL-1, IL-12, IL-18, and tumor necrosis factors (TNFs) and interferon-gamma (IFN-γ), which results in inflammation of tissues [14]. Pro-inflammatory cytokines like IL-6 and IL-1β are released from the macrophages and monocytes in the wound and result in pain responses by signaling the neurons [15]. IFN-γ, IL-1β, and TNF-α induce apoptosis and pyroptosis mediated by the activation of innate immunity and oxidative stress [16]. IFN-γ is an activator; it activates macrophages by stimulating STAT1 expression in order to activate the defense mechanism against the pathogens in the infected area [17]. IL-12 stimulates TNF-α and IFN-γ production and reduces the expression of IL-4, an anti-inflammatory cytokine, and negatively controls the expression of IFN-γ; IL-4 also through the activation of STAT-3 signaling inhibits IFN- γ [18]. IL-18 for defense against pathogens activates T cells and natural killer

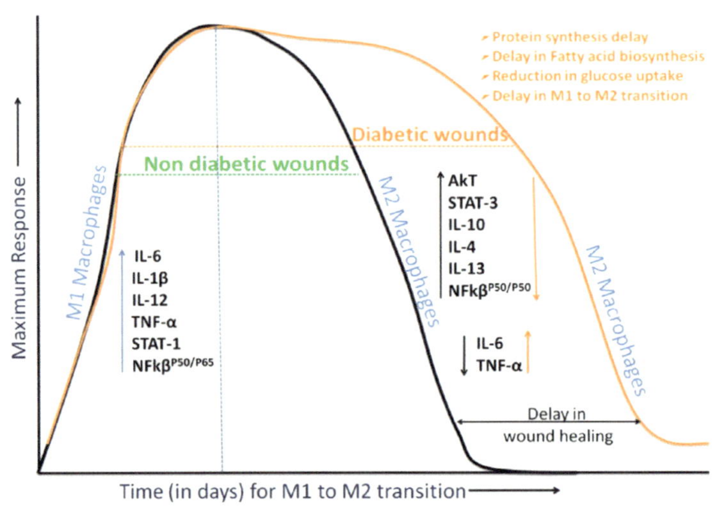

Figure 1.
M1 macrophages (also known as classically activated), such as IL-12, IL-1β, IL-10, STAT1, TNF-α, and NFkβP50/P65, are leads to wound inflammation. Alternatively, active, that is, M2 macrophages, such as STAT3, HIF-α, PKC, NFkβP50/P50, etc., help in healing of the wound by decreasing inflammation. People having diabetes show prolonged M1 macrophage expression in wounds in comparison to nondiabetic wounds that delay M1 to M2 macrophage transition.

(NK) cells and promotes the expression of of IFN-γ cytokines at the wound site [19]. However, the prolonged expression of inflammatory cytokines leads the damage of tissues, which results in a delay in the repairing process of wounds. IL-1 is a TNF activator and is responsible for the damaging of cells. IL-1β overproduction is responsible for neuronal tissue inflammation, leads to damage of neuro-muscular junctions and ultimately leads to delaying in wound healing [20]. In the presence of pathogens, the macrophages secrete IL-6 which in turn increases Toll like receptor expression (TLR)-9 response-mediated defense for killing foreign particles. In case of prokaryotes, unmethylated DNA activates the TLR-9 pathway and helps in killing the pathogen at the wound site; mitochondrial DNA spillage, essentially the unmethylated DNA, triggers similar kind of responses in the tissue of wound [21]. In tissues, the angiogenesis is inhibited by IL-12 by overexpression of IFN-γ-mediated interferon-gamma-induced protein 10 (CXCL-10 or IP-10) [22]. Vascular endothelial growth factor (VEGF) expression is negatively controlled by IL-18, essential for the development of new blood vessels at the wound site and is essential for the growth and repair at wound tissue [23].

To start and control the wound healing mechanism, the inflammation is most important. In the nondiabetic wounds, anti-inflammatory cytokines like IL-4, IL-10, IL-13, IL-11, and transforming growth factor-beta (TGF-β) and interferon-alpha (IFN-α) play an important role in the wound healing process [24]. At the initial stage of wound recovery, TLR-9 induces the instant expression of pro-inflammatory signals like TNF-α through the increase in expression of mitogen-activated protein kinase (MAPK)/p38 and c-Jun N-terminal kinase (JNK) pathway [25]. In non-diabetic wounds, MAPK activation is prolonged and leads to MAPK phosphatase enzyme activation, which works as a negative regulator of JNK and MAPK/p38 pathways, resulting in the negative regulation of TNF-α production. The de-phosphorylation of MAPK/p38 leads to more expression of anti-inflammatory cytokines such as IL-10 a homodimeric cytokine, which is produced by the macrophages, monocytes and induce signaling of TGF-β, and can enhance the division of cells [26]. Cytokines like IL-4, IL-13, and IL-10 can stimulate extracellular matrix and fibrinogen, mainly collagen synthesis. IL-4, cytokines secreted by macrophages, mast cells and inflamed T cells activate the Janus kinase/signal transducer and transcription-6 (Jak/STAT6) pathway activator which promotes the wound repairing [27]. IL-4 is responsible for the extracellular matrix synthesis, mainly collagen which gives the physical support for the healing of the wound [28]. Another kind of cytokine, L-1RA, secreted from immune cells, adipocytes cells and cells of epithelia, leads the inhibition of pro-inflammatory IL1β cytokine effect by binding with the (IL-1R) interleukin-1 receptor. On the other hand, deregulation of TNF-α and IL-1β prolongs the phase of inflammation phase and leads to delay in wound healing [29]. IL-11 released from cells of bone marrow expresses anti-inflammatory effect. IL-11 inhibits the synthesis of IL-1 and TNF-α synthesis by the inhibition of NFkβP50/P65 with increasing the expression of inhibitory NFkβP50/P50 synthesis in monocytes/macrophage cells [30]. Transition between cytokines of pro and anti-inflammatory is balanced in nondiabetic wounds but in case of diabetic wounds, it gets impaired (**Figure 1**).

For the type-1 diabetes treatment or insulin-dependent diabetes, insulin is administrated systematically.

2. Activation of anti-inflammatory cytokines and increased differentiation of cells by signaling through insulin

Insulin, released from pancreatic gland produced in its beta cells of the islets of Langerhans is a peptide hormone. Insulin precursor is proinsulin in humans, is encoded by the INS gene and is a single polypeptide; after processing of proinsulin, two secretory proteins are produced, one chain having two chains namely A (21 amino acids) and B (30 amino acids), which forms mature insulin, and the second is C-chain known as C-peptide having 31 amino acids [31, 32]. Chain "A" is more compact having (2 small) α-helix region; on other hand, B chain has 1 such region. Two disulfide bonds between A20-B19 and A7-B7 hold chain A and chain B together; in addition to this, there is a disulfide bridge between A7-A11 cys amino acids of chain A. In the presence of Zn^{2+} and at ~6.0 favorable insulin pH, it folds to hexameric forms and is stored in pancreas. After diffusion of insulin in blood, with change in the pH, the hexameric insulin form changes to its monomeric form and shows binding with the insulin receptor [33]. The insulin binding with receptors depends on the regions present in the insulin monomeric form. The binding regions are present on the surface of insulin receptors; the changes or mutations in the binding regions reduce the insulin binding affinity [34]. The regions are located at TyrA19, AsnA21, CysA20, on the "A" chain C-terminus, IleA2, GlyA1, GluA4, ValA3, on the N terminus and at PheB24, GlyB23, TyrB26, and PheB25 at B" chain C-terminus (**Figure 2**) [35].

The insulin is found only in the humans, but peptides which are like insulin are also present in invertebrates like insects and molasses. Insulin-like peptides are having growth-related functions, and it indicates that the insulin is not only involved in metabolism of glucose but has other functions as well [37]. Drugs which can balance between the pro-inflammatory and anti-inflammatory cytokines can also be helpful for the treatment of other insulin-independent or dependent diabetes mellitus and its linked disease conditions. Using insulin as a wound-healing agent, very few studies have been found.

The anti-inflammatory effect by insulin is shown by activating the cytokine expression that can decrease the inflammation and help in recovery of the wound. Through metabolism and synthesis activities, insulin shows its effect on the differentiation and survival of cells. Insulin promotes NF-kβP50/P50 upregulation by the suppression of TNF-α and p65 expression. NF-kβP50/P65 expression suppression leads to decrease in expression of proinflammatory cytokines like IL-12, IL-1β, IL-6, and TNF-α cytokines at the site of wound [38]. Proinflammatory cytokine inhibition shifts the equilibrium towards the anti-inflammatory cytokine expression, like

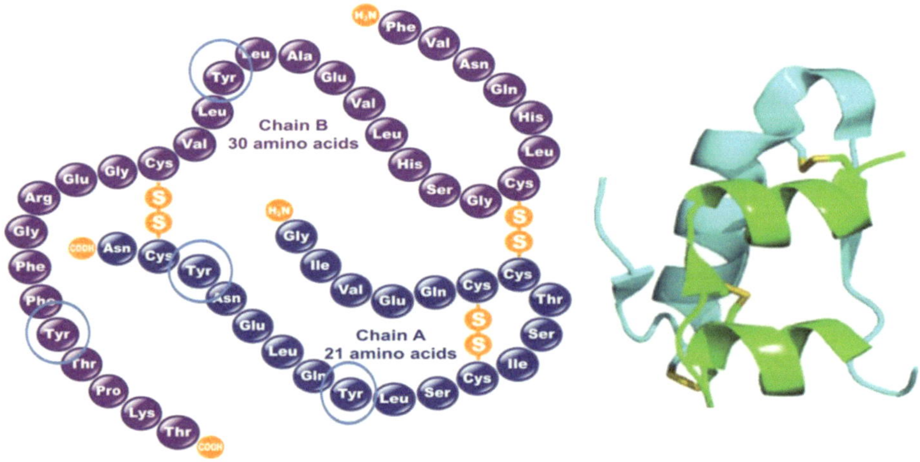

(a) (b)

Figure 2.
Insulin structure (a) showing the sequence of amino acids present in insulin protein (b) showing the 3-D model of insulin [36].

IL-4, IL-10, and VEGF, etc., inhibits the apoptosis of cells, and increases proliferation of cell similarly like IGF [39]. Below sections show the regulation of cytokine dynamics by the insulin: (a) Inactivation of NFkβp50/p65 by insulin results in decrease in inflammation by inducing uptake of glucose uptake, (b) biosynthesis of fatty acid induction by insulin and inactivation through TNF-α, (c) role of insulin in cell differentiation and growth by synthesis of protein and inhibition of proteolysis by inactivation of FOXO to promote the survival of cell, (d) insulin functions like IGF and activates the same signaling pathway and reduces inflammation, and (e) anti-inflammatory action of insulin by reduction in proinflammatory cytokines and increased expression of the anti-inflammatory cytokines (**Figure 3**).

2.1 Role of insulin to promote wound recovery

2.1.1 Inactivation of NFkβp50/p65 by insulin results in decrease in inflammation by inducing uptake of glucose

The presence of high concentration of glucose at the wound site promotes microbial growth and leads to inflammatory signaling activation. The main function of insulin in the body is regulation of blood glucose level. It helps in the utilization of the glucose present in the blood through activation of glucose transporters and stored in glycogen form in the cells. The glycogen stored in the tissue of muscles behaves as a source of energy and gets used aerobically [40]. Wounds mainly in peripheral nerves, renal cortex, and retina are results from microcirculatory damage mainly due to increment in consumption of wound by the inflammatory cells, which leads to switch from aerobic glycolytic to anaerobic glycolytic [41]. The direct result of this is the lactic acid formation as the end glycolysis product. In addition to this, other resources of anaerobic glycolysis are the wound-proliferating cells, which are showing anaerobic respiration in the muscle cells [42]. In the blood, the lactic acid gets used in the liver to form glucose.

Lactate converts into pyruvate and nicotinamide adenine dinucleotide (NADH); NADH behaves as a substrate for nicotinamide adenine dinucleotide phosphate (NADPH) oxidase and helps in the formation of reactive species of oxygen (ROS) induced by lactate [43]. Due to more NADPH synthesis, NADPH to NAD+ ratio

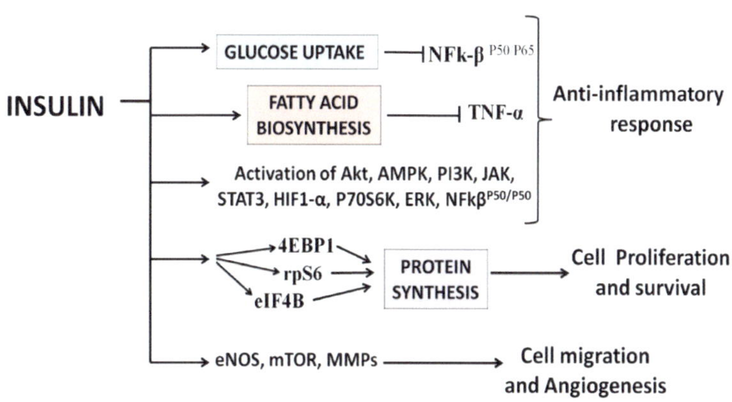

Figure 3.
Insulin plays an important role as an anti-inflammatory agent and helps in the survival of cells by synthesis and metabolic pathways. Glucose metabolism activates NFk-β, and biosynthesis of fatty acids leads to TNF-α activation which can inactivate the inflammatory signaling. By this signaling, insulin helps in the survival of cells and synthesis of protein. Along with this, the insulin activates the Akt pathway and can increase mTOR, MMPs, and eNOS expression leading to the formation of new blood vessels. Insulin can also decrease the NFkβP50/P65 expressions by the ERK and MEK pathways like the pathway for glucose uptake.

reduces, which leads to the VEGF activation and angiogenesis. NADPH and pyruvate, both lead to the formation of new blood vessels and collagen through the inactivation of prolyl hydroxylase hypoxia inducible factor (HIF PHD) [44].

HIF causes the damage of tissue and inflammation at the wound [45]. Hypoxia is also responsible for the damage of peripheral blood vessels and also causes activates NADP oxidase (NOX) to generate oxidative stress in the wound, regulating key factor in the process of wound recovery and leading to inter-cellularly ROS overexpression [46]. High ROS level induces oxidation of protein and peroxidation of lipid, which causes apoptosis of cells [47]. The production of ROS leads to accumulation of NFkβP50/ P65 and inhibits HIF1 α and mTOR expression. In addition to mTOR and HIF1 inhibition, NFkβp50/NFkβp65 induces resistin expression, and both are responsible for intercellular insulin resistance [48]. The resistin leads to the activation of vicious cycle through p65 overexpression [49]. P65 activation shifts the equilibrium from NFκβp50/p50 to NFκβp50/p65 and results in insulin resistance generation [50]. It also induces mTOR and HIF1, by activation of the AKT pathway and inhibition of TNFα [51]. HIF1 activation shifts back to NFκβp50/p65 to NFκβp50/p50 equilibrium. The blood glucose normalization is possible with insulin proper functioning and also by the effective reduction of NFkβP50/P65 expression [52]. NFkβP50/P50 activation reduces expression of proinflammatory cytokines like IL-6 and IL-1β, induces high anti-inflammatory cytokine expression, leads to reduction in inflammation stage, and enhances repairing of tissue [50].

Pyruvate and NADPH inactivate the expression of HIF PHDs, by the oxidation of ascorbic acid and Fe (II). HIF PHDs are the dioxygenase and are 2-oxoglutarate and Fe (II)-dependent and require ascorbic acid. In lactate presence, ascorbic acid and Fe (II) get oxidized and inhibit damage of tissue and increase IL-8release, basal fibroblast growth factor (bFGF) and NF-kβP50/P50 activation [53]. Lactate also upregulates the expression of NF-kβP50/P50 by suppressing the formation of NF-kβP50/P65 and results in reduction of expression of IL-12, IL-1β, TNF-α, and IL-6 cytokines. This pathway ultimately results in more cell viability. Also, ROS-dependent IkBɑ expression inhibition and VEGF receptors are responsible for synthesis of collagen and angiogenesis [54]. IkBɑ helps in NFkβ translocation from nucleus, and p65 gene expression in turn is responsible for inflammation [55]. Along with this, NF-kβP50/P65 expression suppression happens through the phosphorylation of ERK through signaling of insulin [56]. In contrast to these findings, the lactate formed in skeletal muscles impairs the signaling of insulin and results in glucose metabolism inhibition [57]. Glucose metabolism signaling of insulin occurs through 6-phosphofructo-1-kinase (PFK-1), which in turn is formed by pyruvate dehydrogenase (PDH) and fructose-2, 6-biphosphate and used for the conversion pyruvate to oxaloacetate. This signaling of insulin is inhibited by lactate through the production of more citrate and reducing fructose-2, 6-biphosphate, and inhibits and promotes PFK-1 expression, respectively. Inhibition of PDH by rising ratio of NADH to NAD ultimately stops the pyruvate to oxaloacetate transformation [58]. This negative effect of lactate on glucose metabolism shows that it acts as an glycolysis inhibitor and results in increase in concentration of glucose in the blood serum [59]. The glucose high concentration in the blood leads to long-time expression of the inflammation cytokines at the wound site (**Figure 4**).

2.1.2 Fatty acid biosynthesis induction by insulin and inactivation through TNF-α pathway

Insulin also plays different other functions like it can stimulate the synthesis of protein and lipogenesis, as well as differentiation and growth of cells [60]. The lipogenesis is the fatty acid synthesis process which converts acetyl-CoA to triglycerides [61]. Lipogenesis is stimulated by insulin through two types of enzyme activation, PDH (pyruvate dehydrogenase), responsible for pyruvate conversion to acetyl CoA and another acetyl CoA carboxylase helps in conversion of acetyl to malonyl CoA. In the cytoplasm, Malonyl CoA gives 2-C building blocks, used for larger fatty acid synthesis [62]. Transportation of acetyl CoA from mitochondria to cytoplasm occurs by tricarboxylate translocase enzyme, after formation of citrate by reaction with oxaloacetate. The glucose shows a role in increasing the release of both citrate and insulin [63].

Fatty acids, mainly polyunsaturated, play an important role in the formation of cell membrane. Cell membrane composition affects the absorption of enzymes which are responsible for cell phosphatidylinositol 4-kinase (PI4K) proper functioning; membrane associated phosphatidylinositol kinase shows an important role in signaling of cell [64]. The fat metabolism products activate PI4K, which in turn regulates the Protein Kinase C (PKC) functioning and controls proinflammatory cytokine TNF-α signaling [65]. PKC also induces inflammation through increasing the NFkβ and p38MAPK expression. In PI4K presence, the activity of PKC is inhibited, which leads to the reduction of proinflammatory cytokine (TNF-α) release [66]. The free fatty acid component plays an important role in the wound recovery process (**Figure 4**).

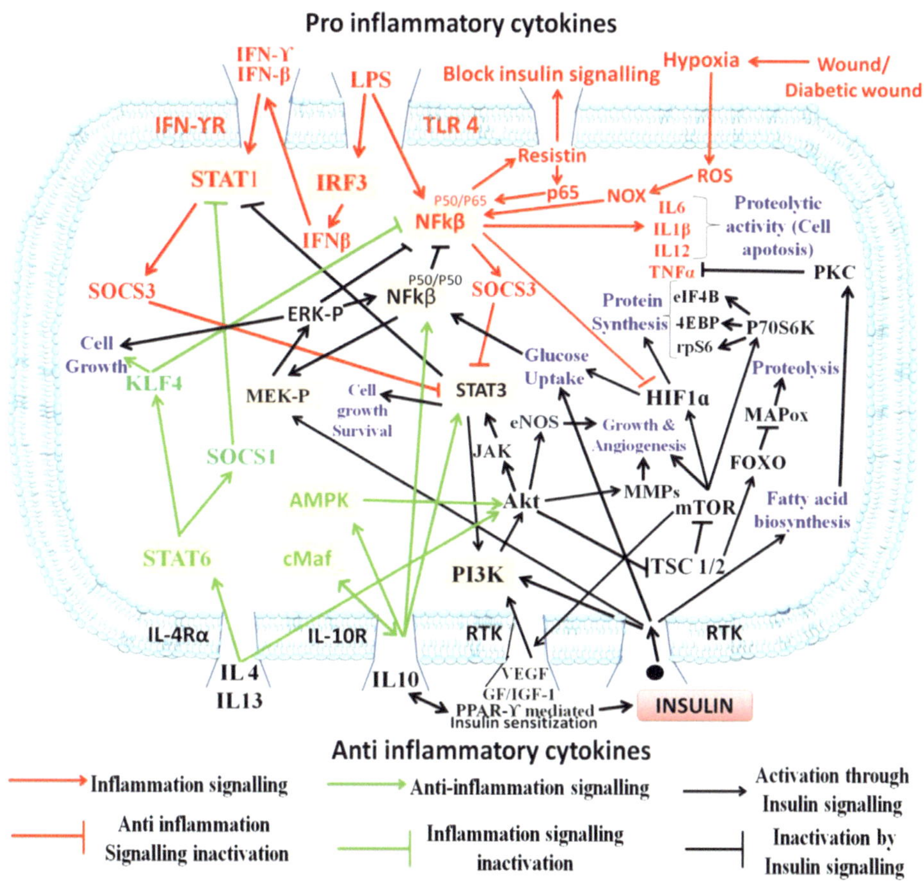

Figure 4.
Transition pathway from M1 to M2 macrophages. TNF α and IFN Υ activate NFk β, STAT1, and IRF-3 at the wound site and help in the release of IL-10, IL-12, NFkβP50/P65, TNF-α, IL-1β, and STAT-1 leading to inflammation. M1 to M2 transition is important for wound recovery. IL-10, IL-4, IL-13, VEGF, insulin, and IGF can activate HIF-α, STAT3, and NFkβP50/P50 cytokines to activate the anti-inflammatory action.

2.1.3 Role of insulin in cell differentiation and growth by synthesis of protein and proteolysis inhibition by the inactivation of FOXO to enhance the survival of the cell and tissue

Insulin stimulates the synthesis of protein in different cells and tissues. In muscle tissues, insulin affects the flow of blood and amino acids uptake by the tissues of muscle and helps in anabolism in the muscles [67]. It has been studied that insulin systematic uptake loses the muscle volume, which mainly happens due to insulin systematic infusion and results in the reduction of the amount of free amino acids in blood and plays an important role in the anabolism in muscles [68]. The deficiency of insulin can be overcome by systematically giving insulin exogenously [69]. Essential protein formation is stimulated by promoting the concentration of RNA contents in the cells and tissues by the insulin functioning pathway through the translocation of the mRNA by the phosphoinositide-3-kinase (PI3K) pathway [70]. By the PI3K pathway, an Akt inhibits the tuberous sclerosis protein ½ (TSC1/2) functioning and behaves like an inhibitor of the mechanistic target of rapamycin (mTOR) and in the end by phosphorylation of 4E Binding protein (4EBP-1leads it activates the eukaryotic initiation factor (eIF4B)). The eukaryotic 2^0 structured mRNA 5'end eIF4B binds. During the synthesis of protein, eIF4B binds with subunits of eIF4A and eIF4G, further binding with ribosome 40S, and it has RNA helicase absent or low results in impairment in the synthesis of protein. The mTOR activation leads to proteolysis inhibition by MAPox activation [71]. High concentration of insulin in the muscle cells inhibits the protein degradation and leads to muscle cell and tissue expansion [72]. Due to inhibition of protein degradation, the insulin ultimately leads to reduce the blood amino acids concentration [73]. This amino acid concentration regulation of insulin clearly indicates that insulin plays a very important part in the diabetic wound healing condition when the patients are on systemic treatment of insulin (**Figure 4**).

2.1.4 Insulin behaves the same as insulin-like growth factor and can also activate similar pathway to decrease the inflammation

Insulin-like growth factor (IGF) is composed of two IGF ligands such as IGF-I and II. At the time of embryogenesis, IGF are the proteins that regulate development and growth, tissue differentiation in adults and show anti-inflammatory actions through the activation of anti-inflammatory cytokines. Insulin shows anti-inflammatory effect by increasing release of IL-10 and IL-13/4. By decreasing pro-inflammatory cytokines release (IFN-ϒ) [74]. IGFs show binding with the insulin receptor (IR), insulin-related receptor, and IGF receptor (IGF-1 and IGF-2). Main functions of IGF-I and II are mediated by Insulin Growth Factor Insulin receptor (IGF-IR) [75]. IGF-I is an important growth factor produced by the macrophages, fibroblast keratinocyte, and platelets. It enhances endothelial cell migration into the wound site. It enhances the mitosis and fibroblast cell proliferation for the new blood vessel formation and extracellular matrix and activation of protein kinase B signaling. In addition to this, it also enhances the synthesis of protein and blocks the muscles atrophy in order to skeletal hypertrophy catalysis [76].

Upon binding with receptor, the IGF-I activates the insulin receptor substrate-1 (IRS-1) which in turn by phosphatidylinositol-4, 5-bisphosphate 3-kinase (PI3K) phosphorylates the protein kinase B (Akt). Phosphorylated Akt activates the mTOR; PI3K-related kinase controls the proliferation of the cells [77]. Also, IGF-I enhances cell growth by activating the mitogen-activated protein kinase/extracellular signal regulated kinase/MAPK/ERK pathway through RAF/RAS kinase phosphorylation of [78]. Along with this, IGF-I binding of receptor enhances the secretion of anti-inflammatory cytokine such as IL-10 activates Akt by AMPK signaling. Likewise, such as IL-4 and IL-10 can also bind with Akt and plays role in M2 macrophages infiltration at the site of wound (**Figure 4**).

2.1.5 The anti-inflammatory action of insulin through a reduction in pro-inflammatory cytokine expression enhances the formation of anti-inflammatory cytokines

The decrease in action of insulin may be due to resistance of insulin or due to the insufficient insulin release, and it ultimately results in diabetes mellitus. The functioning of insulin either reduces due to the β-cells functioning loss or due to the improper functioning of insulin receptors or due to the kidney disease [79]. The insulin treatment systemically is already taken by 6 million people of America, and it keeps on increasing to control high blood glucose condition. High blood glucose concentration leads to the tissue damage by the oxidative stress through increasing flux of other sugars and glucose by the polyol pathway and also enhances the expression end products of advanced glycation and it's activating ligand receptors and through the overexpression of the pathway of hexosamine and activation of protein kinase. The mechanisms mainly take place by the overexpression of mitochondrial ROS [80]. In the polyol pathway, due to more NADPH consumption in the glucose transport pathway, more redox stress is generated and remains insufficient to form the scavengers of ROS that is GSH reduced form advanced glycinated product precursor formation modifies the proteins of plasma that can bind with the receptors of the advanced glycination product present on the surface of macrophages, smooth cells and vascular endothelial cells. This activation of NFkβ transcription factor, in turns activates HIF-α and results in hypoxia stimulated chemokines production through the ROS production [81]. In the presence of high glucose, the protein kinase enzyme shows hyperactivity and stimulates the expression of eNOS in the smooth muscles cells and leads to the destruction of tissue. Increased ROS expression shows the activation of different proinflammation pathways and helps in generating the epigenetic changes, which can result in the prolonged expression of the proinflammatory genes during the wound recovery. Matrix metalloproteinase (MMP-2, 4) excessive production impairs the recovery process of wound and results in extracellular matrix protein breakdown such as vitronectin and fibronectin [82].

In nondiabetic wounds, the wound healing process involves the activation of the series of different physiological events for wound recovery like inflammation at wound site, cell proliferation, epithelisation of cells, vascularisation, maturation, and re-modeling at the site of wound [83]. Macrophages play an important role in the whole healing process. At early wound phase, in the wound recovery process, macrophages function by the cytokine release and activation of leucocytes, which leads to the production of inflammatory response at the site of the wound [84].

The infiltration of the macrophage at the wound site takes place by the effect of chemotaxis which induces the factors like Toll-like receptor (TLR) ligand, PAMP (pathogen-associated molecular patterns), LPS (lipopolysaccharide), PDGF, and IFN-gamma (IFN-ϒ) [85]. M1 macrophages lead to high level secretion of STAT1 and expression of TNF-α or IFN-β. By the activation of the Akt/PI3 pathway, insulin stimulates STAT3, which inhibits STAT1 formation and activates the transition from M1 macrophages to M2 macrophages for the repairing of wound and tissue repairing. M2 macrophages can help in the production of polyamines and ornithine by the pathway of arginase enzyme and anti-inflammatory pathway IL-10, IL-13and IL-4 cytokines [86]. Insulin along with M2 macrophages activates the anti-inflammatory cytokines by Akt, or IP3K pathway activates biosynthesis of protein to induce fatty acid and blood vessel formation and division and migration of cells, to increase wound recovery. With resistance of insulin in diabetic condition, there is constant increase in concentration of proinflammatory cytokines TNFα and IL-6 have been shown in the figure. In the non-diabetic/normal glycemic condition, cytokines are produced by adipocytes such as IL-13, which can promote the M2 activation or alternative macrophages. Alternatively, M2 or activated macrophages are important for the expression of anti-inflammatory cytokine secretion such as IL-10 and PPAR-ϒ (Peroxisome Proliferator-Activated Receptor Gamma) and insulin-sensitizing factors, forming a vicious circle for the functionality of insulin. PPAR-ϒ also activates anti-inflammatory IL-10 cytokine [87] (**Figure 4**).

In the glycemic condition, there is an excessive proinflammatory macrophage expression of cytokines like TNF-α and IL-1β leading to impaired wound recovery. Overactivation of cytokines like IL-17, TNF-α or IL-1β reduces expression of inflammatory cytokines and upregulates genes responsible for wound healing and increases the healing process [86]. In the blood and adipose tissue, the high TNF-α cytokine concentration and TNF-α neutralization improve the insulin sensitivity in the humans or animals. High glucose condition stimulates changes in the gene expression and adipocyte metabolism and lipolysis increment and synthesis of fatty acids (FFAs) and proinflammatory cytokines induces the expressions of macrophages, like tumor necrosis factor α (TNF-α) and monocyte chemotactic protein-1 (MCP-1). M1 macrophage activation produces an excessive concentration of cytokines responsible for inflammation such as TNFα, resistin, and IL-1β, which can act on the cells of adipocyte to make them insulin-resistant. This signaling pathway forms the feedback loop which can increase the resistance to insulin and inflammation [88].

TNF-α, an inflammatory cytokine, performs role in the healing of nondiabetic wound process, but activation of TNF-α for a long time leads to enhancing enzymatic activity of protease enzyme. In human diabetic wounds, MMPs are found in very high amount. In chronic or diabetic wounds, there is imbalance in the expression of cytokines causes proinflammation and their proteases, inhibitors, and their ant protease expression [89].

The switching of macrophages in the high glucose condition gets delayed due to MMPs, IL-1β, IL-6, and ROS cytokine oxidative stress (**Figures 5** and **6**). This leads to delay in M1 to M2 transition and is responsible for the inflammation for long time and leads to delay in the wound recovery [90, 91]. The insulin role in the switching from inflammatory state to anti-inflammatory state is shown in **Figure 5**.

2.1.6 The insulin-like activity of C-peptide

C-peptide consists of only 31 amino acids, is a short peptide and has glycine amino acid-rich regions and behaves like a linker between the two peptides of proinsulin A and B [93]. By ERK1/2 activation and Akt phosphorylation, C-peptide shows angiogenesis. The angiogenesis signaling pathway shows similarity with the VEGF pathway and leads to the formation of nitric oxide by eNOS activation. C-peptide plays a curious role in the cell mitogenesis like insulin, by the same signaling pathway as the insulin protein [94]. C-peptide shows binding to the insulin receptor (IR) and results in intracellular substrate phosphorylation in Ras/MAPK. The PI3K/Akt signaling results in cell division and mitogenesis. Along with the abovementioned two functions, C-peptide also shows its anti-inflammatory effect. C-peptide shows MIP-1a, IL-8, MIP-1β, and IL-6 expression inhibition and other pro-inflammatory cytokine expression [95]. Like insulin, C-peptide can also reduce the problems linked with diabetes, such as vascular inflammation, neuropathy, and nephropathy, in diabetes case especially type 1 diabetes case [96].

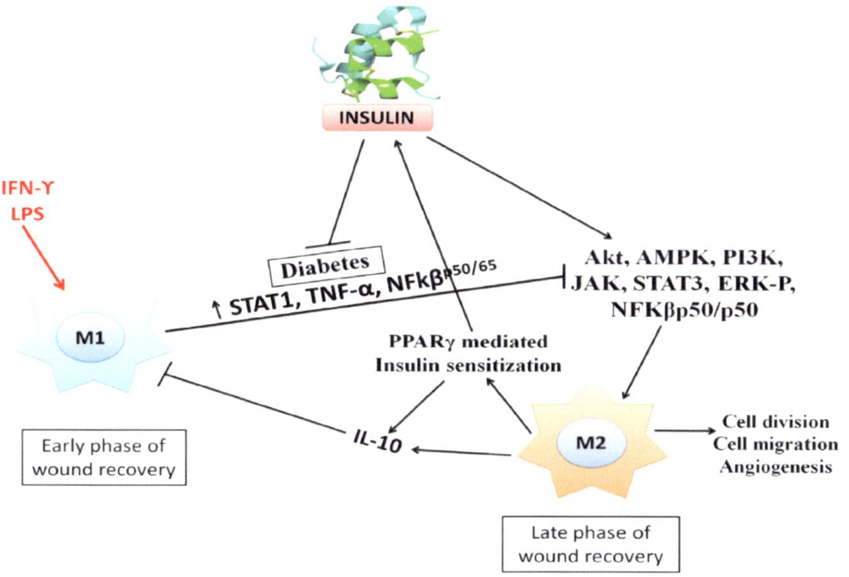

Figure 5.
Effect of insulin on switching of M1 to M2 macrophages. In insulin presence, (AMPK, Akt, STAT3, PKC, HIF-α, PI3K, NFkβP50/P50, and ERK) M2 macrophage expression increases show an anti-inflammatory effect and help in wound healing.

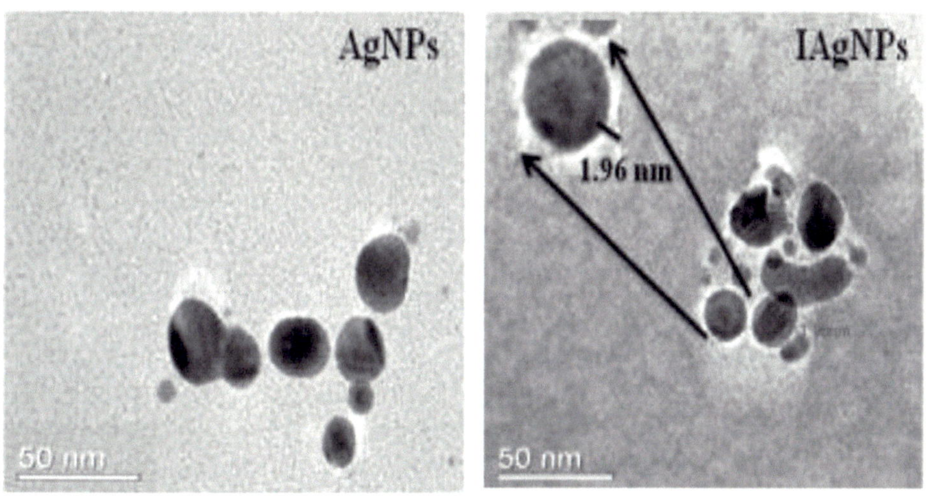

Figure 6.
TEM micrographs of AgNPs and IAgNPs shown with insulin protein coating; the size of AgNPs shifts from around 22 ± 2 to 1.96 ± 0.1 nm. Scale bar: 50 nm [40].

The C-peptide level rises in the blood during diabetic mellitus type 2, which is due to resistance of insulin [97]. At this time, endothelial dysfunction initiated led by the C-peptide deposition in the blood vessel intima walls. The C-peptide deposition causes more inflammation in the blood vessels of the aortic arch and promotes atherosclerotic lesions. The inflammation effect of C-peptide is shown due to C-peptide chemotactic behaviour towards macrophages responsible for inflammation. Monocytes/T-lymphocytes/macrophages migrate through the vessel walls and then release TNF-α, IL-6, and MIF etc., pro-inflammatory cytokines and chemokines and nitric oxide, and activates intracellular signaling pathway [98].

3. Insulin encapsulated mettalic nanoformulations for wound recovery

Nanoparticles of metals such as silver nanoparticles can be used for the delivery of insulin at the site of a wound. Silver nanoparticles have clinical applications due to its antibacterial, anti-inflammatory, and wound healing role. Due to the presence of charge on the surface of metal nanoparticle surface, they are highly reactive and can be surfaces modified by adsorbing different molecules or drugs. The drugs having thiol or amine can easily adsorb on the surface of silver nanoparticles, and due to this, it can help as a drug delivery agent. The anti-inflammatory effect and wound healing (non-diabetic and diabetic) efficiency of silver nanoparticles can be improved by encapsulating the insulin with silver nanoparticles [99, 100].

3.1 Synthesis and characterization of metal insulin nanoparticles

It is very easy to synthesize silver nanoparticles by using reducing and stabilizing agents. Plant extracts like tulsi leaf extract may be used as both reducing and stabilizing agents. The tulsi (*Ocimum tenuiflorum*) aqueous extract of leaves (ATE) was extracted by boiling 3 g of tulsi leaves in water (100 ml for 2 h). After extraction, the extract was allowed to cool and filtered, and the pH of the extract was adjusted to 7.4, and the pH adjusted extract was stored at 4°C for further use. AgNP synthesis was performed by using ATE as a reducing and capping agent. $AgNO_3$ 240 μM was added in ATE (5000 μl) and for 10 min was kept under sunlight. The solution color changed from faint light yellow to reddish brown in the presence of sunlight. After this, AgNPs were incubated with insulin at physiological conditions, the temperature being 37°C for an hour in an incubator in order to produce insulin-protected AgNPs (IAgNPs).

Surface plasmon of nanoparticles with or without protein was monitored using a UV–visible spectrophotometer equipped with Peltier, which showed a resonance peak observed at 352 nm due to the silver nitrate reduction by ATE in sunlight. After incubation with insulin, a blue shift (3 nm) with almost peak intensity double was observed, and λmax was obtained at 349 nm due to the formation of monodispersed IAgNPs. The hydrodynamic size of 22 ± 2 and 42 ± 2 nm (approximately diameter) are observed for AgNPs and IAgNPs, respectively. The Zeta potential showed an increment in the potential values from −12.4 to −15.1 mV due to the conversion of AgNPs to IAgNPs. TEM micrographs showed that both AgNPs and IAgNPs are similar in shape (spherical in shape). AgNP have a size ranging between 20 ± 4 nm, and further, it received a cap of 2 ± 0.5 nm when coated with insulin (IAgNPs) as shown in **Figure 6**.

3.2 Metallic insulin nanoformulation wound healing and anti-inflammatory effect

Wound recovery is promoted by both insulin and IAgNPs in hyperglycemic/diabetic and normal/nondiabetic animal conditions. In both in vivo and in vitro cases, the insulin promotes the wound healing in hyperglycemic and normal conditions. With IAgNPs 12 and 20%, faster wound recovery on treatment's 5th day of the wound was found for nondiabetic and diabetic rats in comparison to the untreated control. Whereas in relation to the IAgNPs, faster wound recovery was shown by free insulin with lesser efficiency with an enhanced rate of 7.27 and 4.67%, respectively, for the normoglycemic and diabetic rate in comparison to untreated rats. The % was 60.0 and 73.33% and with IAgNPs and 33.33 and 40% with only insulin in nondiabetic and diabetic models, respectively, on the 11th day, in comparison to the untreated controls as shown in **Figure 7**.

The quantification of serum showed an increase in anti-inflammatory cytokine percentage and reduction in the expression of inflammatory cytokines in diabetic and normal/normoglycemic animals after treatment with insulin and IAgNPs in comparison to their respective controls. On 5th day, in diabetic rats, the IL-6 concentration was 25%, and TNF-α is in double higher concentration than the normoglycemic control. With treatment of IAgNPs, 50% inhibition of expression of cytokine is much higher than free insulin in both the groups. On the 11th day, IL-6 expression and TNF-α was 30% and 50%, respectively, in control than in normal models, which reduces to 45% in both hyperglycemic and normal animals after treatment with free insulin, and with IAgNPs, the inhibition was around 30% in TNF-α and 40% in IL-6. In addition to reduction in inflammatory cytokine expression, the anti-inflammatory cytokine percentage (IL-10) increases after treating with free insulin and IAgNPs. On the 5th day, IAgNP-treated rats showed that IL-10 increased 50% in diabetic rats and 70% in normal and similarly showed increment in IL-10 concentration of 30% and 45% in diabetic and normal models, respectively, in free insulin-treated groups in comparison to control. On 11th day with IAgNPs anti-inflammatory cytokine concentration was increased by 50 and 65% and with insulin slightly less in both hyperglycemic and normal animals models, respectively. On the 5th and 11th days, the histological evaluations significantly decreased leukocyte infiltration level; faster collagen deposition and fast re-epithelization were observed with insulin and IAgNPs in relation with sub-group (**Figure 8**).

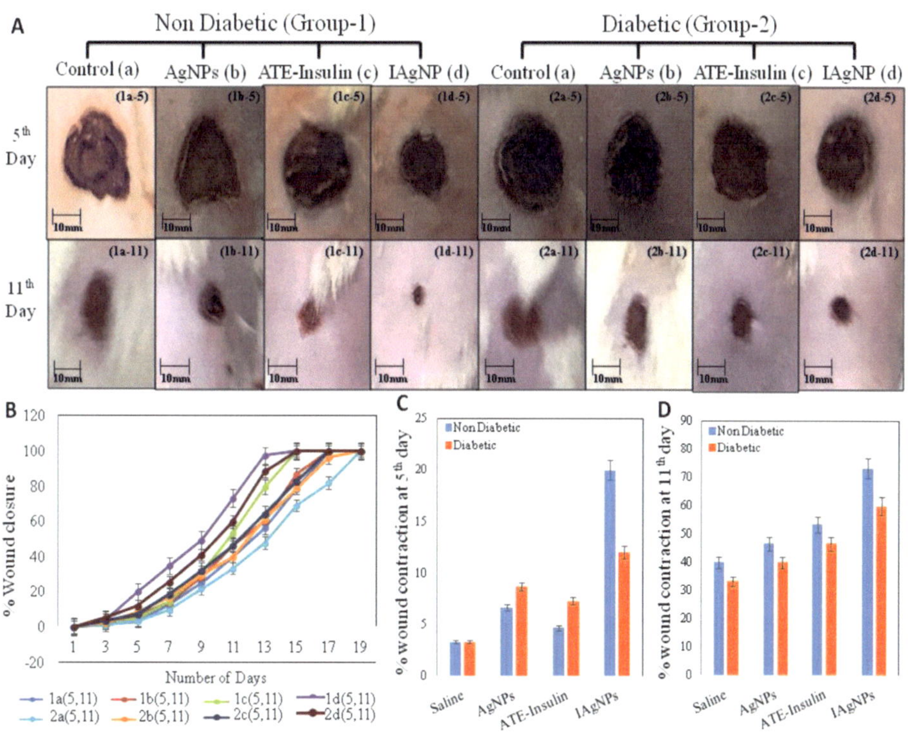

Figure 7.
Wound healing rate of AgNP, ATE-insulin and IAgNP treatment in both hyperglycemic and normal animals on 5th day and 11th day. (A) Wound contraction physical observation in various treatment and control groups. (B) Percentage of closure of wound in different treated groups (AgNPs, ATE-insulin, and IAgNPs) and respective controls of hyperglycemic and normal animals until complete healing of wound takes place. (C) Percentage of contraction of wound in four subgroups of hyperglycemic and normal animals on 5th day. (D) Percentage of contraction of wound in all the four subgroups of hyperglycemic and normal animals on the 11th day [40].

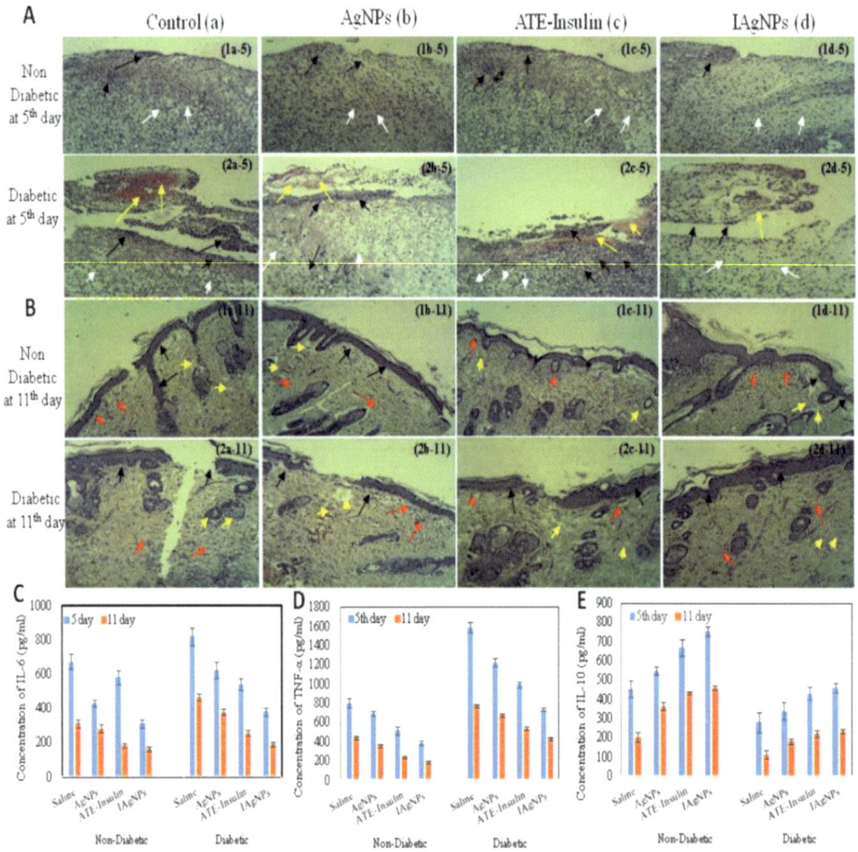

Figure 8.

Histological evaluation (40×) wound site of different groups (a and B, respectively). On the 5th and 11th day of post-treatment, infiltration of leukocyte, formation of exudates and deposition of collagen are denoted by red, yellow and white arrows respectively. Each micrograph represents an overall pattern of a 6-rats group. (C–E). Pro-inflammatory cytokines such as IL-6 and TNF-α and the anti-inflammatory cytokines like IL-10 concentration in all sub-groups of hyperglycemic/and normal animals at 5th and 11th day. TNF-α and IL-6 results show a significant reduction and IL-10 increment by IAgNP treatment in comparison to control, AgNPs, and ATE-insulin-treated animals of both sets on the 5th and 11th day, respectively. Values are shown by the average ± SD of group of six rats [40].

4. Conclusions

Insulin, a hormone which shows the various multiple functions in the body like controlling the inflammation, enhancing the differentiation of cells, biosynthesis of protein and lipid, etc., in addition to controlling the level of glucose in blood through metabolism of glucose. By the metabolism of glucose, the NFkβP50/P50 and IL-8 get activated, causing an inactivation of the IL-1β, TNF-α, NFkβP50/P65, IL-6, resistin IFN- ϒ, and NOX pro-inflammatory cytokines. The metabolism of fat by insulin through inactivating TNF-α mediated pathway also inactivates the pro-inflammatory cytokines. The synthesis of protein gets induced by insulin through Akt; PI3K pathway helps in survival of the cell through the formation of 4EBPI, ribosomal protein S6 (rpS6). This indicates that along with maintaining the blood glucose level, the insulin also shows its anti-inflammatory effect, though the mechanistic aspects of the insulin's anti-inflammatory role is still remained to be elucidated and understood. In addition to biosynthesis and metabolism, insulin pathways have the similarity in structure with IGF-I, can also bind with receptor of IGF and can shows anti-inflammatory activity through PI3K and Akt signaling pathway, which leads to the activation of the pro-inflammatory cytokines such as STAT-3 and can activate Akt again and promote the formation of blood vessels and increases the eNOS production. Likewise, due to similarity in structure, insulin can bind with the receptors of IGF and activate the same pathway as GF/IGF-I, necessitating further studies on insulin, IGFs and their role in anti- response of inflammation (**Figure 5**). About 5% of the world population is diabetic and are in the risk of nonrecoverable or slow wound recovery. The insulin can increase the recovery of wound by inflammatory dynamics modulating, therefore insulin-like inflammatory modulators (such as IGF) or insulin novel formulations based on and have a huge potential for the different clinical applications such as including the diabetic care and should be explored for the beneficiary purposes.

5. Future perspective

Inflammatory regulation is one of the most important factors for wound recovery which caught attention lately. Here in this chapter, the authors have discussed the role of inflammatory regulators in controlling wound recovery taking insulin as an example and model drug for diabetes treatment where wound recovery get delayed to prolonged inflammation. Macrophages in the wound tissue play a critical role in controlling the wound recovery process. Macrophage plasticity is curtailed in the initiation of tissue regeneration, tissue remodeling, and epithelization. Anti-inflammatory activators which can promote M1 to M2 Macrophage transition have a great influence in the promotion of wound recovery. Therefore, anti-inflammatory molecules can be of great virtue for designing advanced wound recovery agents in the future.

Acknowledgements

Diptiman Choudhury is thankful to the DST/SERB project (ECR/2016/000486) for funding. Pawandeep Kaur is thankful to DST inspire, Govt of India, for inspire fellowship under inspire scheme (Award No. IF160636).

Conflict of interest

The authors declare that there is no conflict of interest.

Author details

Pawandeep Kaur and Diptiman Choudhury*
School of Chemistry and Biochemistry, Thapar Institute of Engineering and Technology, Patiala, Punjab, India

*Address all correspondence to: diptiman@thapar.edu

References

[1] King H et al. IDF diabetes atlas: Global estimates for prevalence of diabetes mellitus and impaired glucose tolerance in. Diabetes Care. 1993;**16**:157-177

[2] Harding JL. Global trends in diabetes complications: A review of current evidence. Diabetologia. 2018;**62**:3-16

[3] Wang Y et al. Relationship of diabetes with renal dysfunction in hypertensive adults. Medicine. 2017;**96**:e7169

[4] Baynest HW. Classification, pathophysiology, diagnosis and management of diabetes milletus. Journal of Diabetes & Metabolism. 2015;**6**:2155-6156

[5] Lechner J et al. The pathology associated with diabetic retinopathy. Vision Research. 2017;**139**:7-14

[6] Giacco F, Brownlee M. Oxidative stress and diabetes complications. Circulation Research. 2010;**107**: 1058-1070

[7] Duff M et al. Cutaneous manifestation of diabetes mellitus. Clinical Diabetes. 2015;**33**:40-48

[8] Qing C. The molecular biology in wound healing & non-healing wound. Journal of Trauma and Acute Care Surgery. 2017:323-355

[9] Simo R et al. Neuro degeneration in an early event in diabetic retinopathy: Therapeutic implications. The British Journal of Ophthalmology. 2012;**96**:1285-1290

[10] Patel S et al. Mechanistic insight into diabetic wounds: Pathogenesis, molecular targets and treatment strategies to pace wound healing. Biomedicine & Pharmacotherapy. 2019;**112**:108-615

[11] Tang Y et al. Proresolution therapy for the treatment of delayed healing of diabetic wounds. Diabetes. 2013;**62**:618-627

[12] Gouin JP, Kiecolt Glaser JK. The impact of physiological stress on wound healing: Methods and mechanisms. Immunology and Allergy Clinics of North America. 2011;**31**:81-93

[13] Clark JD et al. Autoinflammatory and autoimmune contributions to complex regional pain syndrome. Molecular Pain. 2018;**14**:1-13

[14] Rachel M et al. Analysis of serum interleukin IL-1β and IL-18 in systemic lupus erythematosus (SCLE). Frontiers in Immunology. 2018;**9**:1250

[15] Laudisi F et al. Cutting edge: The NLRP3 inflammasome links complement mediated inflammation and IL-1β release. Journal of Immunology. 2013;**191**:1006-1010

[16] Lamkanfi M, Dixit VM. Mechanism and function of inflammasomes. Cell. 2014;**157**:1013-1022

[17] Xiao Y et al. Synergestic activation of inflammatory cytokine genes by interferon-ϒ induced chromatin remodelling and toll like receptor signaling. Immunity. 2013;**39**:454-469

[18] Rigante D. The board ranging panorama of systematic autoinflammatory disorders with specific focus on acute painful symptoms and hematologic manifestations in children. Mediterranean Journal of Hematology and Infectious Diseases. 2018;**10**:e2018067

[19] Bernardo ME, Fibbe WE. Mesenchymal stromal cells: Sensors and switchers of inflammation. Cell Stem Cell. 2013;**13**:392-402

[20] Zhang JZ et al. Mitochondrial DNA induces inflammation and increases TLR9/NF-κB expression in lung tissue. International Journal of Molecular Medicine. 2014;**33**:817-824

[21] Sorensen WE et al. IL-2 suppresses vascular endothelial factor receptor 3 expression on tumor vessels by distinc IFN-ϒ dependent mechanisms. Journal of Immunology. 2010;**184**:1858-1866

[22] Lee EY et al. CXCL10 and autoimmune diseases. Autoimmunity Reviews. 2009;**8**:379-383

[23] Harsoliya MS et al. Toxicity of Lps and Opa exposure on blood with different methods. Webmed Central. 2011;**2**:WMC001696

[24] Ma TY et al. TNF-α induced increase in intestinal epithelial tight junction permeability require NFkβ activation. American Journal of Physiology. Gastrointestinal and Liver Physiology. 2004;**286**:367-376

[25] Lappas M et al. Mitogen activated protein kinase proteins regulate LPS-stimulated release of pro-inflammatory cytokines and prostaglandins from human gestational tissues. Placenta. 2007;**28**:936-945

[26] Vieira IR et al. TLR 9 stimulation induces increase in fungicidal activity of human dendritic cells challenged with *Paracoccidioides brasiliensis*. Journal de Mycologie Médicale. 2017;**56**:911-915

[27] Duan XZ et al. Decreased numbers and impaired function of circulating dendritic cell subsets in patients with chronic hepatitis B infection. Journal of Gastroenterology and Hepatology. 2005;**20**:234-242

[28] Kucukcelebi A et al. In vivo characterization of interleukin-4 as a potential wound healing agent. Wound Repair and Regeneration. 1995;**3**:49-58

[29] Dinarello CA. Immunological and inflammatory functions of interleukin-1 family. Annual Review of Immunology. 2009;**27**:519-550

[30] Sultani M et al. Anti-inflammatory cytokines: Important immuno regulatory factors contributing to chemotherapy induced gastrointestinal mucositis. Chemotherapy Research and Practice. 2012;**2012**:11

[31] Kimmel JR, Pollock HG. Studies of human insulin from non diabetic and diabetic pancreas. Diabetes. 1967;**16**:687-694

[32] Huang L. Zinc and its transporters, pancreatic β-cells and insulin metabolism. Vitamins and Hormones. 2014;**95**:365-390

[33] Haeusler RA et al. Biochemical and cellular properties of insulin receptor signalling. Nature Reviews. Molecular Cell Biology. 2018;**19**:31-44

[34] Ward CW et al. The insulin receptor changes conformation in unforeseen ways on ligand binding: Sharpening the picture of insulin receptor activation. BioEssays. 2013;**35**:945-954

[35] Alberto M et al. The chemokines system in diverse forms of macrophages activation and polarization. Trends in Immunology. 2004;**25**:677-686

[36] (a) Human insulin. Stylized chemical structure. (b) PDB 4iyf biological assemblies and structure analysis Protein

[37] Rezvani O et al. A randomized, double blind, placebo controlled trial to determine the effects of topical insulin on wound healing. Ostomy/Wound Management. 2009;**55**:22-28

[38] Hrynyk M, Neufeld RJ. Insulin and wound healing. Burns. 2014;**40**:1433-1446

[39] Azevedo FF et al. Insulin topical modulates inflammatory phase and the angiogenesis of the burns wound healing in diabetic induced rats. Diabetology and Metabolic Syndrome. 2015;**7**:A259

[40] Kaur P et al. Novel nano-insulin formulation modulates cytokine secretion and remodelling to accelerate diabetic wound healing. Nano. 2018;**15**:47-57

[41] Choi J et al. Soluble CD44 is cytotoxic to trabecular meshwork and cells in vitro retinal ganlion. Glaucoma. 2005;**46**:214-222

[42] Price WA et al. Pro-and anti-inflammatory cytokines regulate insulin-like growth factor binding protein production by fetal rat lung fibroblasts. American Journal of Respiratory Cell and Molecular Biology. 2002;**26**:283-289

[43] Gould GW et al. The glucose transporter family: Structure, function and tissue specific expression. The Biochemist. 1993;**295**:329-341

[44] McMillan DE. The microcirculation in diabetes. Microcirculation, Endothelium, and Lymphatics. 1984;**1**(1):3-24

[45] Li Q et al. Insulin regulates glucose consumption and lactate production through reactive oxygen species and pyruvate kinase M2. Oxidative Medicine and Cellular Longevity. 2014;**2014**:504-953

[46] Hajjar DP, Gotto AM Jr. Biological relevance of inflammation and oxidative stress in the pathogenesis of arterial diseases. The American Journal of Pathology. 2013;**182**:1474-1481

[47] Kennedy KM et al. Tumor metabolism of lactate: The influence and therapeutic potential for MCT and CD147 regulation. Future Oncology. 2010;**6**:127-148

[48] Grenz A et al. Hypoxia signaling during intestinal ischemia and inflammation. Current Opinion in Critical Care. 2012;**18**:178-185

[49] Zgheib C et al. Long non-coding RNA lethe regulates hyperglycemia induced reactive oxygen species production in macrophages. PLoS One. 2017;**12**(5):e0177453

[50] Zeng T et al. Blocking nuclear factor-kappa B protects against diet-induced hepatic Steatosis and insulin resistance in mice. PLoS One. 2016;**11**(3):e0149677

[51] Li L et al. Identification of dynamic molecular network in peripheral blood mononuclear cells in type-1 diabetes mellitus. Diabetes, Metabolic Syndrome and Obesity: Targets and Therapy. 2019;**12**:969-982

[52] Steppan CM, Lazar MA. Resistin and obesity associated insulin resistance. Trends in Endocrinology and Metabolism. 2002;**13**:18-23

[53] Liu T et al. NFκB signalling in inflammation. Signal Transduction and Targeted Therapy. 2017;**2**:17023

[54] Paolo EP et al. Lactate stimulates angiogenesis and accelerates the healing of superficial and ischemic wounds in mice. Angiogenesis. 2012;**15**(4):581-592

[55] Backert S et al. Lactate stimulates endothelial cell migration. Wound Repair and Regeneration. 2006;**14**:321-324

[56] Zgheib C et al. Long noncoding RNA lethe regulates hyperglycemia induced reactive oxygen species production in macrophages. PLoS One. 2017;**12**(5):e0177453

[57] Wang Y et al. Artemisinin inhibits monocyte adhesion to HUVECs through the NF-κB and MAPK pathways *in vitro*. International Journal of Molecular Medicine. 2016;**37**:1567-1575

[58] Lovejoy J et al. Insulin resistance in obesity is associated with elevated basal lactate appearance following intravenous glucose and insulin. Metabolism. 1992;**41**:22-27

[59] Guo X et al. Glycolysis in the control of blood glucose homeostasis. Acta Pharmaceutica Sinica B. 2012;**2**:358-367

[60] Saltiel AR et al. Insulin signalling pathways regulating translocation of GLUT4. Nature. 2005;**5**:159-165

[61] Wu M et al. Antidiabetic and antisteatotic effects of the selective fatty acid synthase (FAS) inhibitor platensimycin in mouse model of diabetes. Proceedings of the National Academy of Sciences of the United States of America. 2011;**108**:5378-5383

[62] Murphy MP. Modulating mitochondrial intracellular location as a redox signal. Science Signaling. 2012;**5**:39

[63] Ellen L et al. Selective superoxide generation within mitochondria by the targeted redox cycler mitoparaquat. Free Radical Biology and Medicine. 2015;**89**:883-889

[64] James S et al. Fluid shear stress inhibits TNF-α activation of JNK but not ERK1/2 or p38 in human umbilical vein endothelial cells: Inhibitory crosstalk among MAPK family members. Proceedings of the National Academy of Sciences of the United States of America. 2011;**98**:6476-6481

[65] Adolfo RAP et al. c-Fos activates and physically interacts with specific enzymes of the pathway of synthesis of polyphosphoinositides. Molecular Biology of the Cell. 2011;**22**:4716-4725

[66] Laurence H et al. Signaling pathways involved in LPS induced TNFalpha production in human adipocytes. Journal of Inflammation Research. 2010;**7**:1

[67] Greenhaff PL et al. Disassociation between the effects of amino acids and insulin on signaling, ubiquitin ligases, and protein turnover in human muscle. American Journal of Physiology. Endocrinology and Metabolism. 2008;**295**(3):595-604

[68] Bagry HS et al. Metabolic syndrome and insulin resistance perioperative considerations. Anesthesiology: ASA. 2008;**108**:506-523

[69] Bell JA et al. Short term insulin and nutritional energy provision do not stimulate muscle protein synthesis if blood amino acid availability decreases. American Journal of Physiology. Endocrinology and Metabolism. 2005;**289**:999-1006

[70] Prodhomme M et al. Insulin and amino acids both strongly participate to the regulation of protein metabolism. Current Opinion in Clinical Nutrition & Metabolic Care. 2004;**7**:71-77

[71] Proud CG. Regulation of protein synthesis by insulin. Biochemical Society Transactions. 2006;**34**:213-216

[72] Vijayakumar A et al. Biological effects of growth hormone on carbohydrate and lipid metabolism. Growth Hormone & IGF Research. 2010;**20**:1-7

[73] Guo JY et al. Activated Ras requires autophagy to maintain oxidative metabolism and tumorigenesis. Genes & Development. 2011;**25**:460-470

[74] Higashi Y et al. IGF-1, oxidative stress and atheroprotection. Trends in Endocrinology and Metabolism. 2010;**21**:245-254

[75] Werner H et al. Similarities and differences between insulin and IGF-I: Structures, receptors, and signalling pathways. Archives of Physiology and Biochemistry. 2008;**114**:17-22

[76] Ando Y et al. Epidermal growth factor and insulin like growth factor I enhance keratinocyte migration. Journal of Investigative Dermatology. 1993;**100**:633-639

[77] Burks DJ, White MF. Beta cell and function in type 2 diabetes. Diabetes. 2001;**50**:140

[78] Yamada Y et al. Activation of the Akt-mTOR pathway and receptor tyrosine kinase in patients with solitary fibrous tumors. Cancer. 2014;**120**:864-876

[79] Cefalu WT. Insulin resistance: Cellular and clinical concepts. Experimental Biology and Medicine. 2001;**226**:13-26

[80] Vatankhah N et al. Effect of systematic insulin treatment on diabetic wound healing. Wound Repair and Regeneration. 2017;**25**:288-291

[81] Novak ML, Koh TJ. Macrophage phenotypes during tissue repair. Journal of Leukocyte Biology. 2013;**93**:875-881

[82] Falanga V. Advanced treatments for non healing chronic wounds. EWMAJ. 2004;**4**:11-13

[83] McCormick SM et al. Regulation of macrophage, dendritic cell, and microglial phenotype and function by the SOCS proteins. Frontiers in Immunology. 2015;**6**(6):549

[84] Guo SA et al. Factors affecting wound healing. Journal of Dental Research. 2010;**89**:219-229

[85] Thomsen LH et al. Polarization of macrophages in metabolic diseases. Cellular Immunology. 2015;**6**(6):2

[86] Wang N et al. Molecular mechanisms that influence the macrophage M1–M2 polarization balance. Frontiers in Immunology. 2014;**5**:614

[87] Ferreira AE et al. PPAR-g/IL-10 axis inhibits MyD88 expression and ameliorates murine polymicrobial sepsis. Journal of Immunology. 2014;**192**:2357-2365

[88] Chandirasegaran G et al. Diabetes millerus induced oxidative stress, inflammation and apoptosis: A concise review. ECDMR. 2009;**1**:10-17

[89] Zhu X et al. Micro environment and intra cellular metabolism modulation of adipose tissue macrophage polarization in relation to chronic inflammatory diseases. Diabetes/ Metabolism Research and Reviews. 2018;**34**:e2993

[90] Wetzler C et al. Large and sustained induction of chemokines during impaired wound healing in the genetically diabetic mouse: Prolonged persistence of neutrophils and macrophages during the late phase of repair. Journal of Investigative Dermatology. 2000;**115**:245-253

[91] Kasuya A et al. Attempts to accelerate wound healing. Journal of Dermatological Science. 2014;**76**:169-172

[92] Porta C et al. Molecular and epigenetic basis of macrophage polarized activation. Seminars in Immunology. 2015;**27**:237-248. DOI: 10.1016/j.smim.2015.10.003

[93] Jornvall H et al. Oligomerization and insulin interactions of pro-insulin C-peptide: Three folds relationships to properties of insulin. Biochemical and Biophysical Research Communications. 2010;**391**:1561-1566

[94] Bhatt MP et al. C-peptide replacement as an emerging strategy for preventing diabetic vasculopathy. Cardiovascular Research. 2014;**104**:234-244

[95] Haidet J et al. C-peptide reduces pro-inflammatory cytokine secretion

in LPS-stimulated U937 monocytes in condition of hyperglycemia. Inflammation Research. 2012;**61**:27-35

[96] Bloomgarden ZT. Diabetes complications. Diabetes Care. 2004;**27**:1506-1514

[97] Hills CE et al. Cellular and physiological effects of C-peptide. Clinical Science. 2009;**116**:565-574

[98] Walcher D, Marx N. C-peptide in the veaael wall. The Review of Diabetic Studies. 2009;**6**:180

[99] Gunasekaran T et al. Silver nanoparticles as real topical bullets for wound healing. The Journal of the American College of Certified Wound Specialists. 2012;**3**:82-96

[100] Patra CR et al. Targeted delivery of gemcitabine to pancreatic adenocarcinoma using cetuximab as a targeting agent. Cancer Research. 2008;**68**:1970-1978

Chapter 5

Managing Patients with Pressure Ulcers

Eglantina Afonso, Dina Borges, Kátia Furtado, Maria do Céu Marques, Margarida Pedro, Inês Reis and Rita Morais

Abstract

This study describes care for the person and the informal caregiver with pressure ulcers. The qualitative methodological approach was used, and case study research and the data collection techniques used were the semi-structured interview and the questionnaire. The following scales were applied to the patient: Braden Pressure Ulcer Risk Assessment, Resvesch 2.0, Malnutrition Universal Screening Nutritional Assessment. Modified Barthel and direct observation of wounds, use of the acronym Tissues, Inflammation/infection, Moisture, Edges/Epithelium. The nursing intervention at the patient's home was positive in the evolution of the pressure ulcer healing and in the management of the caregiver's emotions. Providing nursing home care to the injured person is a balm for patients and caregivers. It is an excellent response to aging and consequent complications, for example, wounds. They promote gains in health and in the management of human and economic resources.

Keywords: pressure ulcers, home care nursing, caregiver and informal, caregiver burden

1. Introduction

The technological and scientific development of medicine has increased the average life expectancy. Today, living more years is not synonymous with quality of life. Society's increased concern with the perception of the quality of life is not consensual, but its association with health is unanimous.

Health is a state of balance between the physical and the mental, without discomfort and suffering, which enables the individual to function as effectively as possible in the environment, and a change in this balance causes malaise [1]. Nowadays, health policies favor homecare for dependent people [2]. The Development Plan of the National Network for Integrated Continuous Care [RNCCI] reinforces this concept by stating that the community is the most privileged place for patient care and that each person is responsible for their life and their family as a socio-family reference; therefore, home is a key aspect in health care [3].

With the increase in the population age as well as the need for care, new health requirements emerge. The RNCCI has formed Integrated Continuing Care [ECCI] to provide homecare, focusing on dependent people whose situation does not require hospitalization but who cannot move independently and where the focus of care is centered on the patient and the informal caregiver, who are equally involved. This informal care is the care given to dependent people by their family, friends and neighbors [4]. The informal caregiver is undoubtedly a valuable aspect not only for patient care but also for the health teams provided by the state. This alliance requires the informal caregiver to be available as well as to develop caregiving skills. Given this scenario, the challenge of health policies will be to strike a balance between self-care, informal support and care provided by professionals [5].

Despite the growing interest in the positive aspects of care given by the caregiver, there is still some predominance of negative impacts. Home nursing care is a difficult task influenced by different factors [6]. Thus, it is intended that the benefits become the core of the issue. Stimulating the role of the informal caregiver is essential to keep the patient at home, to optimize his quality of life and avoid his institutionalization [7].

Nursing as a science that takes care of the human being is committed to educating and guiding [8], as one of the competences of the general care nurse. As mentioned in article 5, it is the nurse's responsibility to guide and supervise, transmitting information to the patient aiming at changing behaviors for the acquisition of healthy lifestyles or health recovery, following this process and introducing the necessary adjustments [9]. The community nurse has the role of educating by promoting adequate education as well as information and training.

One of the reasons for admitting patients to ECCI is the treatment of pressure ulcers [PUs] and/or wounds, the admission criterion being the existence of an informal caregiver as a help from the home care team, so that continuity of care is guaranteed and to achieve the goals in the prevention and treatment of complex wounds.

Physical dependence leads to long periods of immobility, endangering skin integrity, leading to the appearance of PUs [1]. PUs represent a public health problem, both nationally and internationally. These entail marked economic burdens for a country, hence the growing political and economic concern [10], and are considered the third or fourth most expensive pathology in the world [11]. PUs are an indicator of the quality of health care provided. The personal suffering caused by this pathology affects the quality of life of patients and caregivers, which can lead to death in extreme situations [12].

The European Pressure Ulcer Advisory Panel [EPUAP] in 2014 defined PU as a localized lesion on the skin and/or underlying tissue, usually over a bony prominence, as a result of pressure or a combination of torsion forces [13]. This entity classifies PUs according to their stage of evolution into six categories/grades, as follows: Category/Grade I: non-blanching erythema; Category/Grade II: partial loss of skin thickness; Category/Grade III: total loss of skin thickness; Category/Grade IV: total loss of tissue thickness; non-gradable/unclassifiable: indeterminate depth; and suspected deep tissue injury: indeterminate depth [13].

The appearance of a PU is largely due to an association of the following risk factors, such as immobilization, nutritional status, skin integrity, age and blood oxygenation level. PUs do not only occur in the geriatric population, but they can also occur in any individual who has one or more of the risk factors mentioned [14]. Demographic changes, such as the growth of the elderly population with multiple co-morbidities, lead to an increase in the number of people with injuries [15]; hence, the prevention and treatment are a challenge for health professionals, especially, nurses. According to the DGS Guideline, 95% of PUs are preventable by early identification of the degree of risk [12]. Therefore, the assessment and management of the risk of developing PUs require a general and multidisciplinary approach to the person [16].

This study aims to describe care for the person and informal caregiver with pressure ulcers.

2. Methodology

This study consists of qualitative research, more specifically a case study, with a central focus on the user and the caregiver, who are provided nursing care by the Integrated Continuous Care Team of a city in southern Portugal.

After selecting the patient for the study, informed consent was requested from the legal representative, his wife, since the patient presented changes regarding his orientation of time and space, as evidenced by the application of the Mini-Mental State scale. The study was submitted to the Ethics Committee of the Baixo Alentejo Local Health Unit.

This type of study seeks to relate the evolution of a phenomenon associated with an intervention. For this, the following resources were used: data collection through semi-structured interviews with the informal caregiver and application of the Informal Caregiver Burden Assessment Questionnaire [QASCI]. Regarding the patient, the following were used: application of the Pressure Ulcer Risk Assessment Scale: Braden Scale [12]; application of the Resvech 2.0 Scale; application of the Malnutrition Universal Screening Nutritional Assessment Scale [MUST] [17]; application of the Barthel Modified Scale [18] and direct observation of the PU, through photographic recording and based on the acronym Tissues, Inflammation/infection, Moisture, Edges/Epithelium [TIME]; the data collection through the clinical process of the patient and the diagnostic evaluation according to the life activities following the Roper-Logan-Tierney theoretical model [19], related to the changed daily living activities [DLA] in the patient. For the elaboration of the diagnostic judgments, the language of the International Classification for Nursing Practice [ICNP] [20] was used, based on the Nursing Interventions Classification [NIC 2010] and the Nursing Outcomes Classification [NOC 2010].

3. Results

3.1 Appreciation

The case study was carried out to the AF patient, male, 70 years old, Caucasian, Portuguese nationality, who lives in Beja, with an Elementary School Education, retired, married, and living with his wife and a daughter.

Personal history: hypertension; depressive syndrome; ethanolic habits, cerebral vascular accident (CVA) in 2013 with left hemiparesis, senile dementia, vascular epilepsy, venous insufficiency of the lower limbs, inguinal hernioplasty, pneumonia, acute cholecystitis and urinary tract infection. Once part of the ECCI, the patient presented with four PUs, with three of them already cicatrized (sacred, left shoulder and right trochanter).

Daily medication: ®baclofen 50 mg at breakfast and bedtime; ®warfarin 1.25 mg at 7 pm; ®pantoprazole 40 mg before meal; ®sertraline 50 mg at breakfast; ®enalapril 20 mg at breakfast and ®sodium valproate 500 mg every 8 h.

After the CVA in 2013, the patient started at RNCCI, having integrated three units. On August 11 of 2016, he was admitted in ECCI, referenced by the family health team for wound care at home. During a home visit, on August 12, 2016, four PUs were found instead of one (information given on the first day). For the healing of the sacred PU, there was a need for constant articulation with the family health team and surgery team. During the 27 months with the ECCI, the left trochanter PU did not have the expected evolution, despite its smaller size.

The patient presents with total dependence on ADL, as demonstrated by the Barthel Modified Scale Assessment with a zero score, with ankylosis of the joints, which makes hygiene care and mobilization difficult, maintains home support three times a day (hygiene and transfers). The equipment that exists in the patient's home is an alternating pressure mattress and a shower chair. The patient gets up daily to an armchair and sleeps in a double bed with inadequate equipment. The patient presents with incoherent speech, hydrated and flushed skin and mucous membranes, normal nutritional status, with a body mass index [BMI] of 23.1. The patient has as an informal caregiver his wife, who is less than two years old than the patient, manifesting difficulties in taking care of her husband, presenting with physical and mental stress overload.

To describe the ADL, the theoretical model previously mentioned was used. Regarding his breathing and controlling body temperature, it remained unchanged. Mobilization is compromised in bedridden and ankylosing patients, and they are dependent on transfers and positions. The patient was not supported by the team's physiotherapist since he was already in a rehabilitation unit. His work and leisure time are compromised, due to his illness and dependence. Regarding the alimentation, it is his wife who prepares and feeds him soft diet meals and protein supplements, using a syringe. His wife is concerned about his well-being and quite motivated by the food aspects, which manifest with increased concern.

Personal hygiene and dressing are compromised, being performed by the home support team, with the supervision of the caregiver. Elimination is compromised but without alteration of the bladder and intestinal pattern. Regarding the following: his sleep, sleep habits are maintained; sensations, the patient presented on the observer scale, without pain; integument, compromised with the presence of PU in the left trochanter; memory, patient is disoriented in space, time and himself.

3.2 Analysis and discussion of results

PUs are lesions that require prolonged and difficult treatment. It depends not only on the therapeutic care provided, such as the frequency of treatment and the suitability of the dressing material, but also on the general condition of the patient and the care provided to him or her by the informal caregiver, such as the frequency of positioning/repositioning; adaptive equipment; pressure reduction and relief. Based on the recommendations of NPUAP/EPUAP & PPPIA [13], the supporting surfaces are essential and should be chosen according to the pressure redistribution needs and other therapeutic functions of the individual.

Based on the diagnosis of needs, it is essential to define intervention strategies, to plan the nursing interventions appropriate to the individual, using appropriate assessment instruments.

Concerning the degree of risk of developing PU according to the Braden Scale, the patient's FA has a total score of 13, which represents a high risk, since DGS [12] reports that a score less than or equal to 16 is high risk. According to the DGS [12], the assessment of the risk of developing PU is fundamental for planning and implementing PU prevention and treatment measures. From the application of the instrument to the patient, it is verified that the mobilization and the friction and sliding forces are the most relevant factors that condition the healing of the wounds and the reappearance of new injuries, despite the intervention with the caregiver through the transmitted information and the results and lessons learned: wheelchair acquisition, viscoelastic cushion, articulated bed and correct positioning techniques, and the informal caregiver due to individual and cultural factors did not adhere to the intervention proposals planned by health professionals. The patient has an alternating pressure mattress in the bed and the caregiver positions it without collaboration, however, and uses incorrect positioning techniques, causing damage to tissue already regenerated, as occurred in the sacred region, not considering the guidelines of health professionals.

Regarding the patient alimentation, the caregiver is concerned about the food and water intake of the patient and makes daily protein supplements. In the application of the MUST instrument, the assessment is low risk.

The informal caregiver demonstrates physical and psychological overload, proven by the application of the QASCI instrument (in October and December 2018). Given the scores, it is noteworthy that the caregiver presents instability in the performance of her role as a caregiver. The caregiver's condition worsened in November 2018, when she initiated restrictions on her health, through non-adherence to the therapeutic regimen for arterial hypertension, dental abscesses and osteoarticular pain. The caregiver's imbalance in biological, psychological and social factors has repercussions on the care she gives. ECCI's multidisciplinary team from Beja articulated with the caregiver and family team referring her to a psychiatry consultation, having attended only one consultation.

When the patient had a stroke in 2013, PU appeared, and there was a need for nursing intervention and entry into the ECCI. In the beginning, the left trochanter PU was grade I, and it was aggravated due to the number of hours that the patient remained in the left lateral decubitus, to relieve the existing PU. In the beginning, the treatment applied was once a day with ®hyperoxygenated fatty acid and protection with polyurethane foam with ®sodium carboxymethylcellulose. On September 19, 2016, the UP presented: devitalized tissue, bleeding tissue, without smell, bounded edges, with a dimension of 5 cm [cm] long by 3 cm wide. The treatment applied daily was enzymatic debridement due to the risk of hemorrhage, with irrigation with a solution of ®polyhexamethylene guanidine [PHMB], ®calcium alginate with silver and foam ®polyurethane with ®sodium carboxymethylcellulose. Articulation with the family team was carried out for close control of the international normalized ratio [INR] and respective therapeutic adjustment of the anticoagulant.

On November 14, 2016, the wound presented: hemorrhage in the wound bed, devitalized tissue, granulation tissue and odor. Despite being referred to the emergency department and a surgery doctor, his wife refused to go. Gelatin sponge dressing, pads and patching, dressing and treatment were initiated twice a day, as well as antibiotic therapy after medical observation. On November 20, 2016 (**Figure 1**), there was PU with devitalized granulation tissue, without bleeding, with inflammatory signs (redness and erythema) and without odor. The treatment applied was saline [S], ®carboxymethylcellulose single fibers, polyurethane

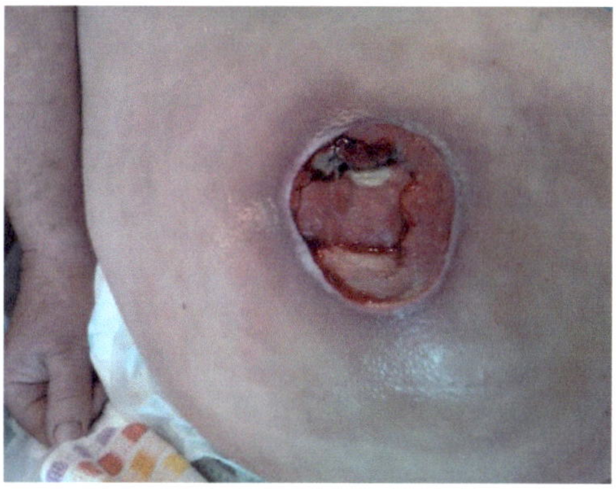

Figure 1.
Left trochanter November 2016, own source.

foam and ®hydrocolloid plate. For a long period, the PU did not evolve, despite vacuum therapy being applied for 1 month, without favorable results due to caregiver resistance. On September 18, 2018, the patient began treatment with honey, ®carboxymethylcellulose single fibers and ®hydrocolloid plaque. In October 2018, the wound did not heal and presented with: devitalized tissue, increased exudate and purulent characteristics, inflammatory signs, and bad smell, the non-healing mnemonics was applied, increased exudate, red and bleeding surface tissue, Dobris [NERDS]. The use of honey was suspended due to the rejection of the informal caregiver; therefore, irrigation with PHMB and carboxymethylcellulose fibers with silver, calcium alginate, polyurethane foam and ®hydrocolloid plate were restarted.

On November 20, 2018, the wound presented: fibrin that was removed, granulation tissue and devitalized, odorless. The treatment was warm saline, ®carboxymethylcellulose single fibers, polyurethane foam and ®hydrocolloid plate (**Figure 2**). Due to acute illness on December 15, 2018 (**Figure 3**), hospitalized patient referred to the unit. He was discharged on January 10, 2019, continuing with ECCI support. On January 23, 2019, PU with granulation and devitalized tissue, macerated and thickened edges, applied with warm saline and

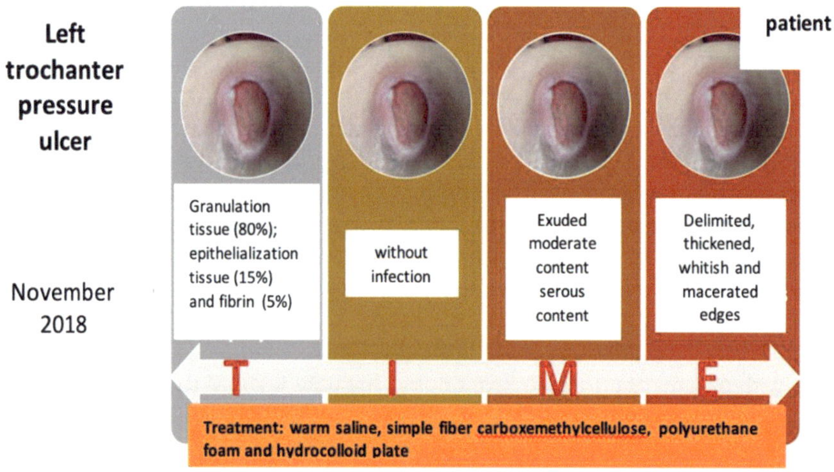

Figure 2.
Evolution with acronym TIME November 2018, own source.

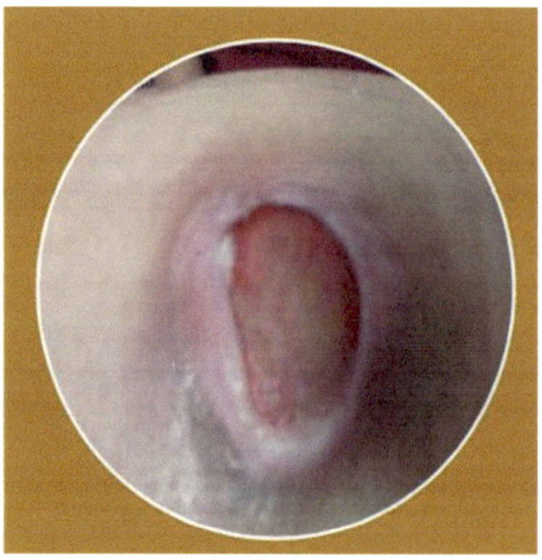

Figure 3.
Left trochanter December 2018, own source.

Date	TIME			
	T	I	M	E
September 19, 2016	Necrotic tissue (10%), devitalized tissue (40%) and granulation tissue (50%)	Pain, redness and edema	Serous hematic and purulent exudate	Delimited edges and macerated perilesional skin
November 14, 2016	Granulation tissue (95%) and devitalized tissue (5%)	Light redness, odor and pain	Considerable sanguineous exudate	Delimited edges
November 20, 2018	Granulation tissue (80%), epithelialization tissue (15%) and fibrin (5%)	–	Moderated serous drainage	Delimited, thickened, whitish and macerated edges
January 23, 2019	Granulation tissue (80%) and devitalized tissue (20%)	Edema, erythema, no odor or pain	Moderated serous drainage	Delimited, thickened and macerated edges

Own source.

Table 1.
Preparation of the wound bed, comparison from August 2016 to January 2019.

®carboxymethylcellulose single fibers, polyurethane foam and ®hydrocolloid plate. For a better understanding, **Table 1** represents the comparison regarding PU bed preparation.

4. Final considerations

We can conclude that a correct diagnosis in favor of the needs felt by the informal caregiver and the patient is crucial in the planning of nursing interventions and the result of health gains for both the patient and those who take care. The positive aspects of the present study were the commitment of the caregiver together with the professionals in self-care in hygiene/comfort and nutrition, leading to the healing of three initial PUs. However, something remained to be done, the barriers created by the caregiver to the management of the physical space, the non-healing of the left trochanter PU and constant maceration of the sacred region, the care inherent in positioning/repositioning avoiding friction and sliding forces, despite the intervention through the teachings done over time. Taking care of a patient is not easy, and the nurse has to know the entire biopsychosociocultural context of the patient and the caregiver, to give the appropriate response to the detected needs. Homecare nurses can promote interventions aimed at favoring and promoting conditions so that the patient and the informal caregiver can transform the negative aspects into positive ones, as a way to achieve a quality of life. What makes the difference is people, for that it is necessary to rethink strategies and put them into practice.

Author details

Eglantina Afonso[1], Dina Borges[2], Kátia Furtado[3], Maria do Céu Marques[4*], Margarida Pedro[5], Inês Reis[1] and Rita Morais[6]

1 Unidade de Cuidados na Comunidade de Beja, Beja, ULSBA, EPE, Portugal

2 Departamento de Enfermagem, Universidade de Évora, Évora, Portugal

3 José Maria Grande Hospital, ULSNA, EPE, Portugal

4 Departamento de Enfermagem, Comprehensive Health Research Centre, Universidade de Évora, Évora, Portugal

5 Vila Real Santo Antonio Community Care Unit, Vila Real de Santo António, Portugal

6 Orthopaedics and Rheumatology Unit, Queen Alexandra Hospital, UK

*Address all correspondence to: mcmarques@uevora.pt

References

[1] Augusto B, Almeida Z. Preservar a integridade Cutânea uma prioridade? In: Ribeiro F, Costa R, Augusto B, Almeida Z, Durão A, Dinis A, Neto I, editors. Feridas e Úlceras Cutâneas. Coimbra: Edições Formasau, Formação e Saúde, Lda; 1999

[2] Andrade FO. Cuidador Informal à Pessoa Idosa Dependente em Contexto Domicílio: Necessidades Educativas do Cuidador Principal (dissertação de mestrado). Universidade do Minho, Instituto de Educação e Psicologia; 2009. Available from: http://repositorium.sdum.uminho.pt/bitstream/1822/10460/1/Disserta%C3%A7%C3%A3o_Mestrado_Fernanda_%20Andrade-Vers%C3%A3o_final.pdf

[3] República Portuguesa. Plano de Desenvolvimento da RNCCI 2016-2019. Ministério da Saúde e Ministério do Trabalho, Solidariedade e Segurança Social; 2016. Available from: https://www.sns.gov.pt/wp-content/uploads/2016/02/Plano-de-desenvolvimento-da-RNCCI.pdf

[4] Ministério do Trabalho, Solidariedade e Segurança Social e Saúde, Portugal. Diário da República. 1.ª Série (N° 24). de 2 de fevereiro de 2017

[5] Lopes L. Envelhecimento Activo: Uma Via para o Bem-Estar. Fórum Sociológico. 2007;**II**(17):65-68

[6] Rice R. Prática de Enfermagem nos Cuidados Domiciliários. Conceitos e aplicações. Lusodidacta: Lisboa; 2004

[7] Cruz D, Loureiro H, Silva M, Fernandes M. As vivências do cuidador informal do idoso dependente. Revista de Enfermagem Referencia. 2010;**III**(2):127-136

[8] Lise F, Silva L. Prevenção de úlceras por pressão: Instrumentalizando a enfermagem e orientando o familiar cuidador. Maringá. 2007;**29**(2):85-89

[9] Ordem dos Enfermeiros. Regulamento do Exercício Profissional dos enfermeiros e Estatuto da Ordem dos Enfermeiros. Lisboa: Ordem dos Enfermeiros; 2012. Available from: http://www.ordemenfermeiros.pt/publicacoes/documents/repe_vf.pdf

[10] Ferreira PL, Miguéns C, Gouveia J, Furtado K. Risco de desenvolvimento de Úlceras de Pressão: Implementação Nacional da Escala de Braden. Lisboa: Lusociência; 2007

[11] Menoita EC. Gestão de Feridas Complexas. Lisboa: Lusodidacta; 2017

[12] Direção Geral da Saúde. Escala de Braden: Versão Adulto e Pediátrica (Braden Q). Lisboa, Portugal: Ministério da Saúde; 2011. Available from: https://www.dgs.pt/departamento-da-qualidade-na-saude/ficheiros-anexos/orientacao_ulceraspdf-pdf.aspx

[13] National Pressure Ulcer Advisory Panel, European Pressure Ulcer Advisory Panel and Pan Pacific Pressure Injury Alliance. In: Haesler E, editor. Prevention and Treatment of Pressure Ulcers: Quick Reference Guide. Osborne Park, Western Australia: Cambridge Media; 2014. Available from: https://sociedadeferidas.pt/documentos/Prevencao_e_Tratamento_de_Ulceras_Por_Pressao-Guia_de_Referencia_Rapido.pdf

[14] Ministério da Saúde. Plano Nacional para a Segurança dos Doentes 2015-2020. Diário da República, 2.ª série N° 28, de 10 de fevereiro de 2018 (Despacho n° 1400-A/2015). Lisboa: Ministério da Saúde; 2015. Available from: https://www.dgs.pt/.../plano-nacional-para-a-seguranca-dos-doentes-2015-2020-pdf

[15] Parreira A, Marques R. Feridas—Manual de boas práticas. Lisboa: Lidel; 2017

[16] Alves P. Úlceras por Pressão: da Ciência Básica à Prática Clínica. In: Parreira A, Feridas MR, editors. Manual de boas práticas. Lisboa: Lidel; 2017

[17] British Association for Parenteral and Enteral Nutrition. Malnutrison Universal Screening Tool. 2010. Available from: http://www.bapen.org.uk

[18] Direção Geral da Saúde. Acidente Vascular Cerebral: Prescrição de Medicina Física e Reabilitação. Lisboa, Portugal: Ministério da Saúde; 2011. Available from: http://www.dgs.pt/directrizes-da-dgs/normas-e-circulares-normativas/norma-n-0542011-de-27122011.aspx

[19] Roper N, Logan W, Tierney AJ. O Modelo de Enfermagem Roper–Logan–Tierney. Lisboa: Climepsi; 2001

[20] Ordem dos Enfermeiros. Classificação Internacional para a Prática de enfermagem; 2010. Available from: http://ordemenfermeirospt/browserCIPE/BrowserCIPE.aspx

Section 2

Hypertrophic Scarring

Chapter 6

Hypertrophic Scarring

Jesus Escriva-Machado, Eduardo Camacho-Quintero, Alejandro Maciel-Miranda, Samuel Almeida-Navarro and Julia De la Luz-Hernandez

Abstract

Hypertrophic scars represent important problems because of the presence of pain, pruritus, contractures, as well as unsatisfactory aesthetic results. Currently, the evidence shows that a multidisciplinary management through prevention, adequate choice of suture, atraumatic surgical technique, and early noninvasive measures can favor the handling of these problems and continue with invasive measures that employ intralesional drugs. Clearly, the combination of surgical, technical, and pharmacological interventions will maximize therapeutic results.

Keywords: hypertrophic scar, scar, pathological scar, surgical scar

1. Introduction

Hypertrophic scars (HS) are defined as a pathological scars that have abnormal thickness and are raised from the previous wound [1]. Such scars are the most common complication of burn injury and abnormal wound healing response after traumatic injury, surgery, or inflammation [2, 3]. These lesions are characterized by their red to purple color, raised appearance, decreased pliability, and tenderness with concomitant symptoms including pruritus and pain [4–9]. Patients with HS may suffer from stiffness, cosmetic disfigurement, joint contractures, as well as impediment in physical function and daily activities, and even psychological issues such as depression or anxiety [1, 10–12].

2. Epidemiology

The best clinical predictor for the development of hypertrophic burn scars is a prolonged inflammatory wound healing phase. This result usually corresponds with a wound that has not epithelialized and continues to exudate for more than 3 weeks [13]. Hypertrophic scars generally develop at about 2 months after a burn and will continue to proliferate for a year or longer. HS maturation may not occur until 18 or even 24 months after a burn. The exact time point of regression or maturation of HS remains unknown [8–10, 14, 15].

According to the literature, about 32–72% of surgical skin wounds result in HS after 1 year [16, 17]. In Asian, the prevalence rate of HS after burn injury is as high as 70%, much higher than in Caucasian populations. Contractures after burns have a prevalence of 38–54% of patients, with up to 46% patients undergoing at least one reconstructive procedure after their acute hospital stays [18, 19] (**Figure 1**).

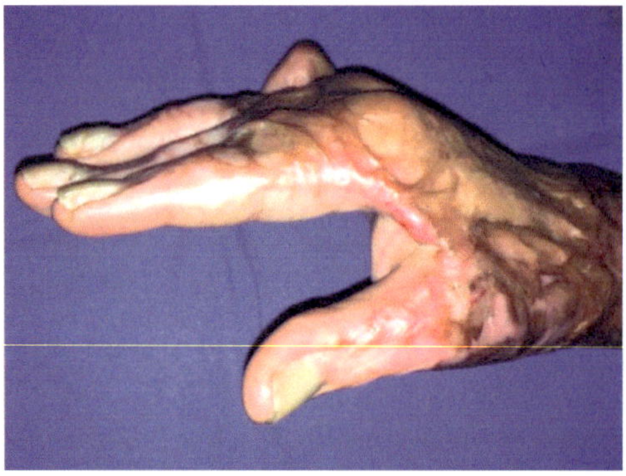

Figure 1.
Patient with a history of flame burn. Hypertrophic scars that affect the first interdigital space.

In order to prevent and treat pathologic wounds, one must first understand the basics of normal wound healing.

3. Wound healing

The desirable result of normal wound healing is replacement of the initial hemostatic clot with skin that approximates the aesthetic, mechanical, and functional properties of the preinjury tissue.

Historically, wound healing has been arbitrarily divided into three phases, with some authors adding hemostasis as the inciting phase. Although wound healing occurs on a time continuum, division of the process into phases allows for ease of description and evaluation. Changes in the steps of normal wound healing may result in either a "hypoplastic" or chronic nonhealing wound or a hypertrophic "over-healed" wound [20].

The clotting cascade is activated immediately after trauma, a consequence of the disruption of the vascular endothelium and exposure of the basal lamina that results in extravasation of blood constituents and concurrent platelet activation. Subsequently, the release of growth factors causes the deposition of extracellular matrix (transforming growth factor β), chemotaxis (platelet-derived growth factor), epithelialization (fibroblast growth factor and epidermal growth factor), and angiogenesis (vascular endothelial growth factor) [21, 22].

4. Inflammatory

An inflammatory phase develops and persists for 4–6 days. This phase is characterized by hemostasis and leukocytic infiltration led by polymorphonuclear leukocytes. Neutrophils, as well as monocytes, fibroblasts, and endothelial cells deposit on a fibrin scaffold formed by platelet activation. The presence of neutrophils is followed closely by monocytes that are quickly activated into tissue macrophages. These cells cause further tissue debridement and secrete additional cytokines as well as growth factors that promote fibroblast proliferation, angiogenesis, and keratinocyte migration [23].

5. Proliferative

The proliferative phase of wound healing begins at 4 days and persists up to 14 days; this phase is heralded by the transformation of monocytes to macrophages.

Keratinocytes initiate epithelialization and are present on the wound edge as well as from dermal appendages such as hair follicles, sweat, and sebaceous glands. Epidermal growth factor, fibroblast growth factor, transforming growth factor β, and multiple cytokines originate cell detachment and mitotic division; then, fibroblasts appear in the wound after 24 hours of this stimulation and produce collagen. This process requires adequate oxygen supply. In fact, without oxygen to assist in the hydroxylation of proline and lysine residues, chemical bonds will not form appropriately to create a mature form of collagen. These bonds are very critical because their absence can prolong the stage and result in a chronic wound. They serve as the basis for the final stage of maturation and remodeling [24].

6. Maturation

Appropriate wound maturation and remodeling result in a quickly healed and minimally visible scar; whereas, prolongation or deviations from this phase can cause hypertrophic, keloid scars or chronic nonhealing wounds. This initial collagen is thinner than uninjured. Type III collagen initially comprises 30% of the granulation tissue matrix, compared with 10–20% in uninjured skin. Over time, the ratio of type III collagen decreases, and type I collagen increases. An overall increase in collagen formation is seen for 4–5 weeks; after this time wound strength increases and parallels the increase in type I collagen [25, 26].

7. Cellular basis, signals and pathways of hypertrophic scars

Fibroblasts and myofibroblasts are pivotal effectors cells in HS [27]. The activation of fibroblasts and differentiation into myofibroblasts (that are a phenotypically intermediate cell type between fibroblasts and smooth muscle cells) are the central processes in the pathophysiology of hypertrophic scars. The larger the area of the wound, the greater migration of myofibroblasts. This situation results in more prominent scarring [28, 29]. Many origins of fibroblasts or myofibroblasts have been characterized: local dermis and subcutaneous tissues around the wound

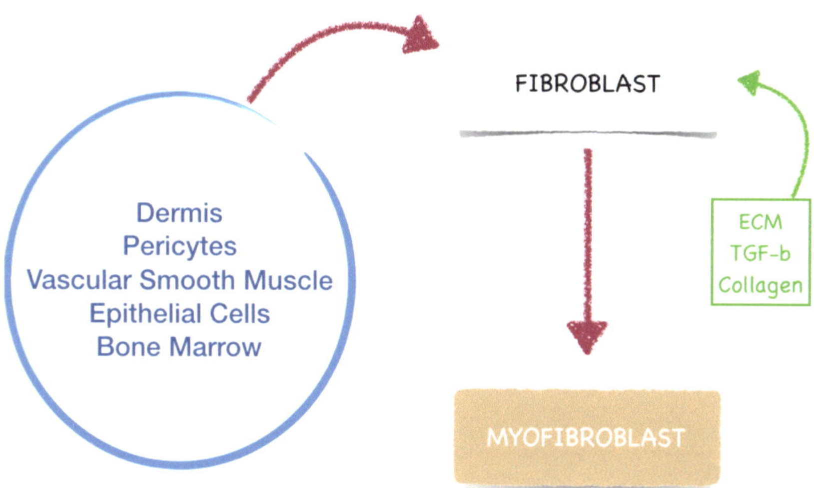

Figure 2.
Activation of fibroblasts and differentiation into myofibroblasts are the central processes in the pathophysiology of hypertrophic scars.

site, pericytes and vascular smooth muscle cells, tubular epithelial cells through epithelial-mesenchymal transition (EMT), tissue specific stem cells, and bone marrow-derived peripheral blood fibrocytes (**Figure 2**) [30].

The proliferative fibroblasts produce massive collagen and make extracellular matrix (ECM) that accumulates below the dermis. One sign thought to be of particular importance is that transforming growth factor-beta (TGF-b), acting through a signaling pathway in fibroblasts, appears to cause an increase in production of ECM and leads to cellular proliferation [31, 32]. Over time, some cells can develop autocrine TGF-b positive feedback loops that can lead to a self-propagating cycle of excessive extracellular matrix production and cell proliferation. Moreover, fibroblasts infiltrate and degrade the fibrin clot by producing matrix metalloproteinases (MMPs) and tissue inhibitor of metalloproteinases (TIMPs). This action results in an imbalance between the formation and degradation of matrix [33].

8. Risk factors

Risk factors for the development of pathologic scarring in the setting of burns have been reported to include darker skin color [1, 34], female sex [35], young age [17, 35, 36], allergy [16, 37], bacterial colonization [38], stretch and burns to the neck or upper limb [35], multiple surgical procedures [35], meshed skin graft [35], increased time to healing [1, 35, 38, 39], and burn depth [35].

Factors that reduce the risk of presenting HS are: chemotherapy [40], smoking [17], statins [41], and genetic background that does not have association [42] (**Table 1**).

Increase HS	
Darker skin color	Stretch
Female sex	Neck and upper limb
Young age	Multiple surgical procedures
Allergy	Meshed skin graft
Bacterial colonization	Increased time healing
Burn depth	
Decrease HS	
Chemotherapy	
Smoking	
Statins	

Table 1.
Overview of factors associated with the development and reduce risk of HS described by other authors to date.

9. Genetic

No convincing evidence exists for a familial pattern in patients who suffer from HS. In a systematic review, the authors did not find any pedigree studies on HS [42, 43].

10. Dark skin

In the literature, dark skin has a higher incidence of HS compared with lighter skin of Caucasians. Dark skin contains more and larger fibroblasts that deposit more collagen, related to what was previously written [1, 34, 36].

11. Female sex

Gangemi and colleagues observed in a multivariate regression model that female sex, young age, burn sites on the neck and/or upper limbs, multiple surgical procedures, and meshed skin grafts were risk factors for postburn pathologic scarring [35].

12. Age

Evidence supports the negative association of age with HS. Excessive scars develop mostly in younger patients between 11 and 30 years old. The inflammatory response decreases with age: epidermal turnover is slower in elderly individuals, and the epidermis contains fewer cells [17, 35, 36, 44].

13. Allergy

Hypothesize that increased degranulation of mast cells observed in allergic individuals supports HS formation. This relationship of allergy with HS formation is supported by level III evidence [16, 37].

14. Bacterial colonization

Bacterial toxins stimulate and prolong the inflammatory phase of wound healing and, thereby stimulate HS [38, 45].

15. Evaluation of hypertrophic scar

Currently no standardized system method exists to assess postsurgical scars. In the literature, scar assessment has mainly been focused on burn scars, but an increasing interest in postsurgical scars is seen, both to evaluate postoperatively as well as to have a closer and objective monitoring when therapeutic measures are applied so as to conclude whether the management is effective or, on the contrary worsening the situation of the scar [4, 9].

Comprehensive scar assessment must include three different dimensions: (a) physical characteristics; (b) cosmetic appearance; and (c) patient's symptoms (**Table 2**).

To date, only four scales have been psychometrically studied: the Vancouver Scar Scale (VSS), the Patient and Observer Scar Assessment Scale (POSAS), the Manchester Scar Scale (MSS), and the Stony Brook Scar Evaluation Scale (SBSES) (**Table 3**).

Scar assessment
Physical characteristics
Cosmetic appearance
Symptoms

Table 2.
Points to scar assessment.

Scar scales
Vancouver scar scale
Patient and observer scar assessment scale
Manchester scar scale
Stony Brook scar evaluation scale

Table 3.
Scales psychometrically studied for the evaluation of scars.

16. Vancouver scar scale (VSS)

The VSS was created in 1990 and is the most widely used rating scale for scars. Four physical characteristics are scored: height, pliability, vascularity, and pigmentation. Each variable is ranked to obtain a total score ranging from 0 to 13, with 0 representing normal skin [46, 47] (**Table 4**).

PIGMENTATION

Normal	Hypopigmentation	Hyperpigmentation
0	1	2

VASCULARITY

Normal	Pink	Red	Purple
0	1	2	3

PLIABILITY

Normal	Soft	Yield	Firm	Band	Contracture
0	1	2	3	4	5

HEIGHT

Normal	<2mm	<5mm	>5mm
0	1	2	3

Table 4.
Vancouver scar scale.

17. Manchester scar scale

The MSS includes six items: contour, texture, color, distortion, shiny surface, and overall patient's opinion [47].

18. Patient and observer scar assessment scale

The POSAS is a recent and promising scar assessment tool that incorporates both observer and patient scar ratings [47, 48].

19. Stony Brook scar evaluation scale

Scars are assigned 0–1 point for the presence or absence of the following: width greater than 2 mm at any point of the scar, raised (or depressed) scar, and darker coloration than surrounding skin. The total score is then derived from the scale and ranges from 0 (worst) to 5 (best) [47, 49].

20. Treatment of hypertrophic scar

Different methods have been described for the treatment of hypertrophic scars. Among those have been found prevention, re-excision with primary closure, massages, compression clothes, silicone sheets, intralesional injections, laser therapy and topical treatments (**Table 5**).

Treatment of hypertrophic scar
No invasive
Prevention
Pressure garment therapy
Scar massage
Laser therapy
Silicone gel sheeting
Invasive
Triamcinolone acetonide
5-Fluorouracil

Table 5.
Treatment of hypertrophic scars.

21. Prevention

The prevention is the conjunction of measures that reduce inflammation and provide rapid wound closure such as early debridement of dead space, reducing the risk of infection through rinsing and disinfection, as well as optimal dressings that provide moist wound healing and/or early surgical wound coverage. During the operation, the surgeon should also use adequate sutures and avoid excessive tension. Surgical closure must be meticulous with an atraumatic technique to generate a successful and minimal linear scar. In the training of plastic surgery, the use of fine and atraumatic instruments is taught for the handling of the tissues for example hooks for retraction. Without a doubt, the tension found in the closure of a wound plays a very important role in widened and hypertrophic scars; these tension forces separate the edges of the wound and generate a wider scar with time. This result can be decreased with the liberation and advancement of the edges, in addition to the placement of correct subdermal sutures [50].

Once the wound has been prepared and is ready for closure, the proper suture and suture technique must be selected. Wounds may be closed with simple interrupted, horizontal mattress, vertical mattress, figure-of-eight, or running sutures. The choice of the suture is of great importance, and most of the time despised, attention should be paid to the estimated time to resorption since the suture may or may not provide adequate support during the healing process. With a Level II of Therapeutic Evidence, polydioxanone (PDS) has been found to result in less scar widening and less scar hypertrophy at 6 months compared with polyglycolic acid (PGA). In the first 3 weeks of wound healing, the strength of a wound is only a small fraction of its eventual strength. Sutures removed or degraded before this time have little effect in preventing wound spreading. Polyglactic acid suture loses strength after 3 weeks, at which time the wound is still relatively weak. These results are similar to removing a nylon suture from the wound in 1 week [51, 52].

Leaving a permanent intradermal suture in place for several months has been shown to decrease spreading, and a synthetic suture possibly retains strength for 6–8 weeks and may have the same effect. This result is caused by the difference in the absorption time and what comes from the loss of tensile strength. On an average PGA scars were wider than PDS scars by 33% (means 9.6, 7.2), the difference that was statistically highly significant (Wilcoxon test $p < 0.001$) [51, 52].

In another study that used the Vancouver Scar Scale (VSS), the scar's width and quality of polydioxanone (PDS) was compared with that of polyglactin 910. The scars were evaluated at 1, 3 and 4 months postoperatively. On follow-up, the mean scar width in Polyglactin 910 was significantly more than that of PDS. The VSS score was significantly lower in the PDS group at the third and fourth month follow up and signified better scar quality [53].

22. Noninvasive measures

22.1 Pressure garment therapy (PGT)

The theory behind the use of PGT may be quite simple and relies on two main concepts; first, the restriction of blood flow to the scar area inhibits the growth of hypertrophic scar tissue and second constant compression does too [54]. Some evidence indicates that PGT may have an effect on the remodeling of hypertrophic burn scar elements such as fibrillin and elastin [55]. In an experimental model with swine that received pressure treatment with a device mounting and delivery at 30 mm Hg of constant pressure for 2 weeks, the total collagen quantification using hydroxyproline assay showed a 51.9% decrease after pressure initiation. Pressure treated scars also had lower levels of collagen I and III after pressure treatment ($P < 0.05$) compared with sham and untreated scars [56]. Using a newly developed pressure therapy system, the Smart Pressure Monitored Suits. Pre and post treatment comparison demonstrated significant improvement in scar pigmentation, thickness, VSS scores, as well as scores of pain and itch ($p < 0.01$) for the early intervention group prescribed within 60 days after injuries compared with the late intervention group prescribed after 61 days. The early group demonstrated superior effect in improving scar lightness, yellowness ($p < 0.01$), thickness ($p < 0.01$), pigmentation score ($p < 0.05$) and pain score ($p < 0.01$) than the late group in comparison between the two groups at similar postburn timing [57].

However, a meta-analysis of clinical results suggests that PGT does not appear to alter global scar scores, but does appear to improve scar height, although this difference is small and of questionable clinical importance. The beneficial effects of PGT remain unproven while the potential morbidity and cost are not insignificant [58].

22.2 Scar massage

Scar massage is used in burn units globally to improve functional and cosmetic outcomes of hypertrophic scarring following a burn; however, the evidence to support this therapy is unknown [59].

22.3 Laser therapy

The three main groups of lasers that can be used to improve scars include pulsed dye lasers (PDLs), Nd:YAG lasers, as well as ablative and nonablative fractional lasers.

A systematic review of the effectiveness of the ablative 10,600 nm CO_2 laser, shows objective improvement in scar color, thickness, and sensation, but not in scar elasticity. All studies reported improvements in the mean total VSS score and/or VSS component scores (pliability, height, vascularity, pigmentation), without statistically significant differences between raters. Statistically significant improvements in both the patient and the observer sections of the POSAS were reported after CO_2 laser treatment. Despite these positive findings, all studies were of low or unclear quality. As a result, insufficient scientific evidence exists to determine the effectiveness of laser therapy for hypertrophic burn scars from this systematic review [60].

22.4 Silicone gel sheeting (SGS)

In 2006, a Cochrane review found weak evidence to support the use of SGS [61]. SGC was effective to reduce thickness, pain, itchiness, and pliability of hypertrophic scars in Chinese the population after 6 month's intervention [62]. Silicone products, either in gel or sheet, are superior to onion extracts including heparin and allantoin in the treatment of the hypertrophic scar [63].

23. Invasive treatment

23.1 Intralesional corticosteroids

In patients with ongoing hypertrophy, more invasive measures are indicated. Intralesional corticosteroids is the only invasive option that has enough supporting evidence [64, 65]. The most commonly used is triamcinolone acetonide (TAC), the dose and treatment interval is variable ranging from 10 to 40 mg/ml given between 2 and 4 weeks interval. The success rate is 50–100% in different studies with 9–50% experiencing recurrence [66, 67]. The TAC injection should be limited to the scar and avoid the periscar tissues. The adverse outcomes of skin atrophy, pigmentation, and telangiectasias are unacceptable by some patients [68–71].

The injection of TAC is not contraindicated in children, but that dose adaption to the child's weight is advised to avoid systemic exposure [72, 73].

Additional injectable treatment options that may help to treat hypertrophic scars (and keloids) include 5-fluorouracil and verapamil.

23.2 5-Fluorouracil (5FU)

The use of antineoplastic agents as treatment options is logical because these abnormal tissues are in hypermetabolic states. 5-FU has been known to affect the fibroblast proliferation in tissue cultures because of its antimetabolite activity and has been shown to be an effective treatment for inflamed hypertrophic scars [28].

23.3 Triamcinolone acetonide and 5FU

This combination is associated with significantly greater reductions in scar size and erythema compared with triamcinolone acetonide alone in a 12-week double-blind study of 40 patients [74]. In a randomized control trial that include 120, patients the mean reduction in scar height was significant in 5FU + TAC group versus TAC alone. Recurrence was seen in 39.2% of patients of the TAC group while in 17.5% of 5FU + TAC group (P = 0.012) [75].

Verapamil is a calcium channel antagonist that both decreases collagen synthesis and increases collagen breakdown. In a randomized, single-blind study of 54 patients with hypertrophic scars or keloids, scar vascularity, pliability, height, and width were reduced with intralesional verapamil, although the rate of reduction in these parameters was slower than with intralesional triamcinolone [76]. A randomized controlled of 50 patients the VSS scores were achieved with no therapeutic event or significant improvement was seen in verapamil group versus TAC group [77].

Pruritus is a chronic problem associated with many hypertrophic scars. Besides the emollient creams mentioned above, the use of local or systemic antihistamines may be useful and depends on the total body surface area involved in the areas of

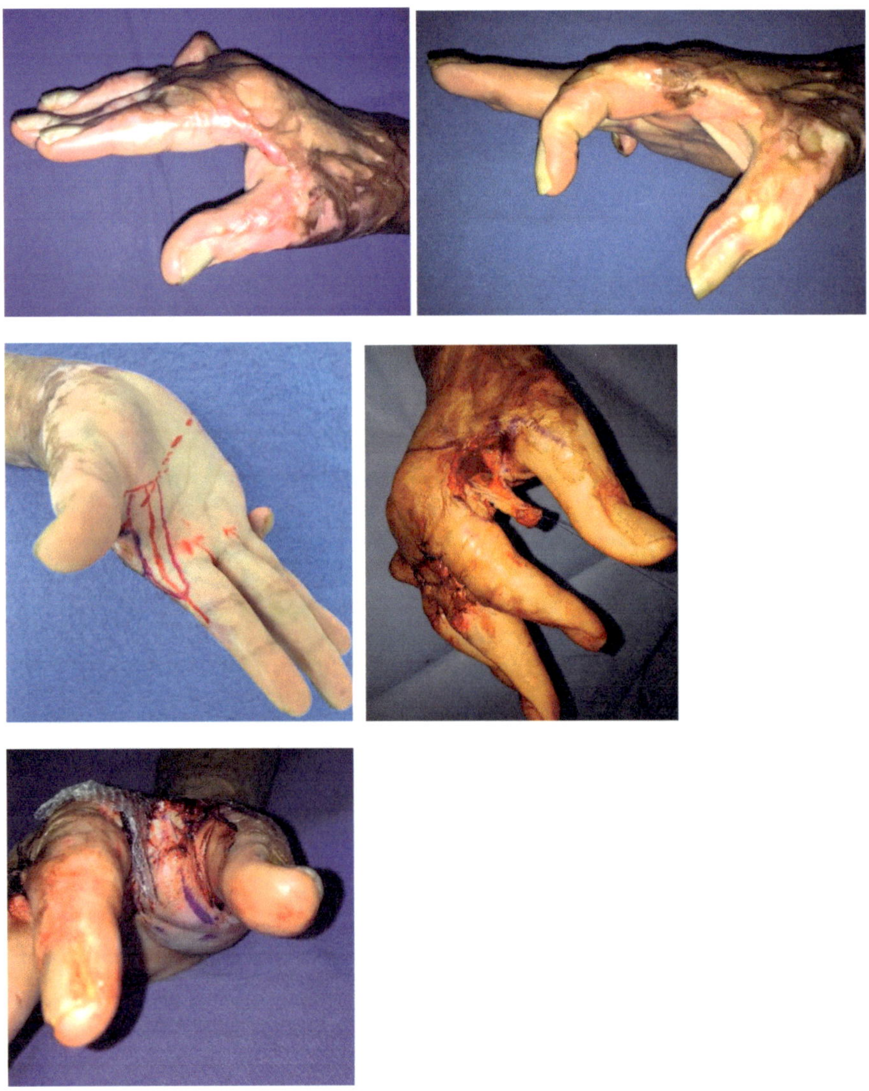

Figure 3.
Release of first interdigital space with flap based on perforating of digital artery of index finger.

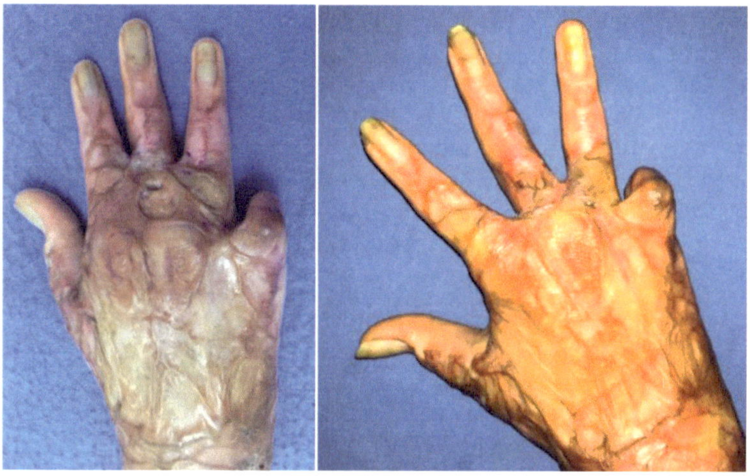

Figure 4.
Multiple syndactyly release in a single time with seagull wings flap.

itchiness. Some early evidence suggests that naltrexone may be a useful treatment for burn-related itching [78].

23.4 Surgical treatment

Surgical interventions for burn scars are usually postponed until the scar is considered "mature" or what may be 6–12 months after maturity, primarily because of the concern of recurrence of the scar. This may also have been influenced by burn scar reconstructive release surgeries performed by grafting and flaps. Most believe that the best option is the treatment with flaps [79] (**Figures 3** and **4**).

Author details

Jesus Escriva-Machado[1]*, Eduardo Camacho-Quintero[2], Alejandro Maciel-Miranda[3], Samuel Almeida-Navarro[1] and Julia De la Luz-Hernandez[1]

1 Puerta de Hierro Tepic Hospital, Tepic, Nayarit, Mexico

2 "20 de Noviembre" Hospital, Mexico City, Mexico

3 Instituto Oncológico Nacional, Guadalajara, Jalisco, México

*Address all correspondence to: jesus.escriva@icloud.com

References

[1] Bombaro KM, Engrav LH, Carrougher GJ, et al. What is the prevalence of hypertrophic scarring following burns? Burns. 2003;**29**(4):299-302

[2] Aarabi S, Longaker MT, Gurtner GC. Hypertrophic scar formation following burns and trauma: New approaches to treatment. PLoS Medicine. 2007;**4**:1464-1470

[3] Wolfram D, Tzankov A, Pülzl P, Piza-Katzer H. Hypertrophic scars and keloids—A review of their pathophysiology, risk factors, and therapeutic management. Dermatologic Surgery. 2009;**35**:171

[4] Bell L, McAdams T, Morgan R, et al. Pruritus in burns: A descriptive study. The Journal of Burn Care & Rehabilitation. 1988;**9**:305

[5] Slemp AE, Kirschner RE. Keloids and scars: A review of keloids and scars, their pathogenesis, risk factors, and management. Current Opinion in Pediatrics. 2006;**18**:396

[6] Anthonissen M, Daly D, Janssens T, Van den Kerckhove E. The effects of conservative treatments on burn scars: A systematic review. Burns. 2016;**42**(3):508-518

[7] Rabello FB, Souza CD, Farina Júnior JA. Update on hypertrophic scar treatment. Clinics (São Paulo, Brazil). 2014;**69**(8):565-573

[8] Nedelec B, Correa JA, de Oliveira A, LaSalle L, Perrault I. Longitudinal burn scar quantification. Burns. 2014;**40**(8):1504-1512

[9] Van den Kerckhove E, Stappaerts K, Fieuws S, Laperre J, Massage P, Flour M, et al. The assessment of erythema and thickness on burn related scars during pressure garment therapy as a preventive measure for hypertrophic scarring. Burns. 2005;**31**(6):696-702

[10] Bock O, Schmid-Ott G, Malewski P, Mrowietz U. Quality of life of patients with keloid and hypertrophic scarring. Archives of Dermatological Research. 2006;**297**(10):433-438

[11] Robert R, Meyer W, Bishop S, Rosenberg L, Murphy L, Blakeney P. Disfiguring burn scars and adolescent self-esteem. Burns. 1999;**25**:581

[12] Taal L, Faber AW. Posttraumatic stress and maladjustment among adult burn survivors 1 to 2 years postburn. Part II: The interview data. Burns. 1998;**24**:399

[13] Matsumura H, Engrav LH, Gibran NS, et al. Cones of skin occur where hypertrophic scar occurs. Wound Repair and Regeneration. 2001;**9**(4):269-277

[14] Ensen LLM, Parshley PFM. Postburn scar contractures: Histology and effects of pressure treatment. Journal of Burn Care & Research. 1984;**5**(2):119-123

[15] Oliveira GV, Chinkes D, Mitchell C, Oliveras G, Hawkins HK, Herndon DN. Objective assessment of burn scar vascularity, erythema, pliability, thickness, and planimetry. Dermatologic Surgery. 2006;**31**(1):48-58

[16] Niessen FB, Schalkwijk J, Vos H, Timens W. Hypertrophic scar formation is associated with an increased number of epidermal Langerhans cells. The Journal of Pathology. 2004;**202**:121e9

[17] Mahdavian Delavary B, van der Veer WM, Ferreira JA, Niessen FB. Formation of hypertrophic scars: Evolution and susceptibility. Journal of Plastic Surgery and Hand Surgery. 2012;**46**:95e101

[18] Chen J, Li-Tsang CWP, Yan H, Liang G, Tan J, Yang S, et al. A survey on the current status of burn rehabilitation services in China. Burns. 2013;**39**(2):269-278

[19] Li-Tsang CWP, Lau JCM, Chan CCH. Prevalence of hypertrophic scar formation and its characteristics among the Chinese population. Burns. 2005;**31**(5):610-616

[20] Gabriel V. Hyperthrophic scar. Physical Medicine and Rehabilitation Clinics of North America. 2011;**22**:301-310

[21] Janis J, Harrison B. Wound healing: Part I. Basic science. Plastic and Reconstructive Surgery. 2016;**138**:9S

[22] Barrientos S, Stojadinovic O, Golinko MS, Brem H, Tomic-Canic M. Growth factors and cytokines in wound healing. Wound Repair and Regeneration. 2008;**16**:585-601

[23] Witte MB, Barbul A. General principles of wound healing. The Surgical Clinics of North America. 1997;**77**:509-528

[24] Kivisaari J, Vihersaari T, Renvall S, Niinikoski J. Energy metabolism of experimental wounds at various oxygen environments. Annals of Surgery. 1975;**181**:823-828

[25] Broughton G 2nd, Janis JE, Attinger CE. Wound healing: An overview. Plastic and Reconstructive Surgery. 2006;**117**(7 Suppl):1e-1S

[26] Ehrlich HP, Krummel TM. Regulation of wound healing from a connective tissue perspective. Wound Repair and Regeneration. 1996;**4**:203-210

[27] Chun Q, Zhiyong W, Fei S, Xiqiao W. Dynamic biological changes in fibroblasts during hypertrophic scar formation and regression. International Wound Journal. 2014

[28] Sarrazy V, Billet F, Micallef L, Coulomb B, Desmouliere A. Mechanisms of pathological scarring: Role of myofibroblasts and current developments. Wound Repair and Regeneration. 2011;**19**(Suppl 1):s10-s15

[29] Curran TA, Ghahary A. Evidence of a role for fibrocyte and keratinocyte-like cells in the formation of hypertrophic scars. Journal of Burn Care & Research. 2013;**34**:227-231

[30] Lian N, Li T. Growth factor pathways in hypertrophic scars: Molecular pathogenesis and therapeutic implications. Biomedicine and Pharmacotherapy. 2016;**84**:42-50

[31] Armour A, Scott PG, Tredget EE. Cellular and molecular pathology of HTS: Basis for treatment. Wound Repair and Regeneration. 2007;**15**:S6-S17

[32] Gabriel V. Transforming growth factor-beta and angiotensin in fibrosis and burn injuries. Journal of Burn Care & Research. 2009;**30**(3):471-481

[33] Ulrich D, Ulrich F, Unglaub F, Piatkowski A, Pallua N. Matrix metalloproteinases and tissue inhibitors of metalloproteinases in patients with different types of scars and keloids. Journal of Plastic, Reconstructive & Aesthetic Surgery. 2010;**63**:1015-1021

[34] Deitch EA, Wheelahan TM, Rose MP, Clothier J, Cotter J. Hypertrophic burn scars: Analysis of variables. Journal of Trauma and Acute Care Surgery. 1983;**23**:895-898

[35] Gangemi EN, Gregori D, Berchialla P, et al. Epidemiology and risk factors for pathologic scarring after burn wounds. Archives of Facial Plastic Surgery. 2008;**10**:93-102

[36] Ketchum LD, Cohen IK, Masters FW. Hypertrophic scars and keloids: A collective review. Plastic and Reconstructive Surgery. 1974;**53**:140e54

[37] Smith CJ, Smith JC, Finn MC. The possible role of mast cells (allergy) in the production of keloid and hypertrophic scarring. The Journal of Burn Care & Rehabilitation. 1987;**8**:126e31

[38] Baker RH, Townley WA, McKeon S, Linge C, Vijh V. Retrospective study of the association between hypertrophic burn scarring and bacterial colonization. Journal of Burn Care & Research. 2007;**28**:152e6

[39] Cubison TC, Pape SA, Parkhouse N. Evidence for the link between healing time and the development of hypertrophic scars (HTS) in paediatric burns due to scald injury. Burns. 2006;**32**:992-999

[40] Lee TJ, Jeong WS, Eom JS, Kim EK. Adjuvant chemotherapy reduces the incidence of abdominal hypertrophic scarring following immediate TRAM breast reconstruction. Breast Cancer Research and Treatment. 2013;**137**:767e71

[41] Ko JH, Kim PS, Zhao Y, Hong SJ, Mustoe TA. HMG-CoA reductase inhibitors (statins) reduce hypertrophic scar formation in rabbit ear wounding model. Plastic and Reconstructive Surgery. 2012;**129**:252ee61e

[42] Bayat A, Bock O, Mrowietz U, Ollier WE, Ferguson MW. Genetic susceptibility to keloid disease and hypertrophic scarring: Transforming growth factor beta 1 common polymorphisms and plasma levels. Plastic and Reconstructive Surgery. 2003;**111**:535e43

[43] Brown JJ, Bayat A. Genetic susceptibility to raised dermal scarring. The British Journal of Dermatology. 2009;**161**:8e18

[44] Enoch S, Price PE. Cellular, molecular and biochemical differences in the pathophysiology of healing between acute wounds, chronic wounds and wounds in the aged. World Wide Wounds. 2004. Available from: http://www.worldwidewounds.com

[45] Edwards R, Harding KG. Bacteria and wound healing. Current Opinion in Infectious Diseases. 2004;**17**:91e6

[46] Sullivan T, Smith J, Kermode J, Mclver E, Courtemanche DJ. Rating the burn scar. The Journal of Burn Care & Rehabilitation. 1990;**11**:256-260

[47] Vercelli S, Ferriero G, Sartorio F, Stissi V, Franchignoni F. How to assess postsurgical scars: A review of outcome measures. Disability and Rehabilitation. 2009;**31**(25):2055-2063

[48] Van de Kar AL, Corion LUM, Smeulders MJC, Draaijers LJ, van der Horst CM, van Zuijlen PP. Reliable and feasible evaluation of linear scars by the patient and observer scar assessment scale. Plastic and Reconstructive Surgery. 2005;**116**:514-522

[49] Singer AJ, Arora B, Dagum A, Valentine S, Hollander JE. Development and validation of a novel scar evaluation scale. Plastic and Reconstructive Surgery. 2007;**120**:1892-1897

[50] Bloemen MC, van der Veer WM, Ulrich MM, van Zuijlen PP, Niessen FB, Middelkoop E. Prevention and curative management of hypertrophic scar formation. Burns. 2009;**35**:463e75

[51] Chantarasak ND, Milner RH. A comparison of scar quality in wounds closed under tension with PGA (Dexon) and polydioxanone (PDS). British Journal of Plastic Surgery. 1989;**42**:687-691

[52] Weinzweig J. Chapter 1: Plastic Surgery Secrets. Second ed. Mosby: Elsevier; 2010. p. 5

[53] Gupta D, Sharma U, Chauhan S, Anand Sahu S. Improved outcomes

of scar revision with the use of polydioxanone suture in comparison to polyglactin 910: A randomized controlled trial. Journal of Plastic, Reconstructive & Aesthetic Surgery. 2018;**71**:1159-1163

[54] Yildiz N. A novel technique to determine pressure in pressure garments for hypertrophic burn scars and comfort properties. Burns. 2007;**33**:59-64

[55] Costa AM, Peyrol S, Porto LC, et al. Mechanical forces induce scar remodeling. Study in non-pressure-treated versus pressure-treated hypertrophic scars. The American Journal of Pathology. 1999;**155**(5):1671-1679

[56] Tejiram S, Zhang J, Travis T, Carney B, Alkhalil A, Moffatt L, et al. Compression therapy affects collagen type balance in hypertrophic scar. Journal of Surgical Research. 2016;**201**:299e305

[57] Li P, Wai Ping Li-Tsang C, Deng X, Wang X, Wang H, Zhang Y, et al. The recovery of post-burn hypertrophic scar in a monitored pressure therapy intervention programme and the timing of intervention. Burns. 2018;**44**:1451-1467

[58] Anzarut A, Olson J, Singh P, et al. The effectiveness of pressure garment therapy for the prevention of abnormal scarring after burn injury: A meta-analysis. Journal of Plastic, Reconstructive & Aesthetic Surgery. 2009;**62**:77-84

[59] Ault P, Plaza A, Paratz J. Scar massage for hypertrophic burns scarring—A systematic review. Burns. 2018;**44**:24-38

[60] Zuccaro J, Ziolkowski N, Fish J. A systematic review of the effectiveness of laser therapy for hypertrophic burn scars. Clinics in Plastic Surgery. 2017;**44**:767-779

[61] O'Brien L, Jones D. Silicone gel sheeting for preventing and treating hypertrophic and keloid scars (review). Cochrane Database of Systematic Reviews. 2006;**1**:CD003826

[62] Li-Tsang C, Lau J, Choi J, Chan C, Jianan L. A prospective randomized clinical trial to investigate the effect of silicone gel sheeting (Cica-Care) on post-traumatic hypertrophic scar among the Chinese population. Burns. 2006;**32**:678-683

[63] Karagoz H, Yuksel F, Ulkur E, Evinc R. Comparison of efficacy of silicone gel, silicone gel sheeting, and topical onion extract including heparin and allantoin for the treatment of postburn hypertrophic scars. Burns. 2009;**35**:1097-1103

[64] Middelkoop E, Monstrey S, Teot L, Vranckx JJ, editors. Scar Management Practical Guidelines. Maca-Cloetens; 2011. p. 1e109

[65] Mustoe TA, Cooter RD, Gold MH, et al. International clinical recommendations on scar management. Plastic and Reconstructive Surgery. 2002;**110**:560e71

[66] Niessen FB, Spauwen PH, Schalkwijk J, Kon M. On the nature of hypertrophic scars and keloids: A review. Plastic and Reconstructive Surgery. 1999;**104**:1435e58

[67] Nanda S, Reddy BS. Intralesional 5-fluorouracil as a treatment modality of keloids. Dermatologic Surgery. 2004;**30**:54-56

[68] Al-Attar A, Mess S, Thomassen JM, Kauffman CL, Davison SP. Keloid pathogenesis and treatment. Plastic and Reconstructive Surgery. 2006;**117**:286e300

[69] Ketchum LD, Smith J, Robinson D, Masters FW. The treatment of hypertrophic scar, keloid and scar

contracture by triamcinoloneacetonide. Plastic and Reconstructive Surgery. 1966;**38**(3):209-218

[70] Friedman SJ, Butler DR, Dittelkov MR. Perilesional linear atrophy and hypopigmentation after intralesional corticosteroid therapy. Journal of the American Academy of Dermatology. 1988;**19**:537-541

[71] Jucket G, Hartman-Adams H. Management of keloids and hypertrophic scars. American Family Physician. 2009;**80**:253e60

[72] Sclafani AP, Gordon L, Chadha M, Romo T III. Prevention of earlobe keloid recurrence with postoperative corticosteroid injections versus radiation therapy: A randomized, prospective study and review of the literature. Dermatologic Surgery. 1996;**22**:569e74

[73] Patel PA, Bailey JK, Yakuboff KP. Treatment outcomes for keloid scar management in the pediatric burn population. Burns. 2012;**38**:767e71

[74] Darougheh A, Asilian A, Shariati F. Intralesional triamcinolone alone or in combination with 5-fluorouracil for the treatment of keloid and hypertrophic scars. Clinical and Experimental Dermatology. 2009;**34**:219e23

[75] Khalid F, Mehrose M, Saleem M, Yousaf M, Mujahid A, Rehman S, et al. Comparison of efficacy and safety of intralesional triamcinolone and combination of triamcinolone with 5-fluorouracil in the treatment of keloids and hypertrophic scars: Randomised control trial. Burns. 2019;**45**:69-75

[76] Margaret Shanthi FX, Ernest K, Dhanraj P. Comparison of intralesional verapamil with intralesional triamcinolone in the treatment of hypertrophic scars and keloids. Indian Journal of Dermatology, Venereology and Leprology. 2008;**74**:343e8

[77] Abedini R, Sasani P, Mahmoudi H, Nasimi M, Teymourpour A, Shadlou Z. Comparison of intralesional verapamil versus intralesional corticosteroids in treatment of keloids and hypertrophic scars: A randomized controlled trial. Burns. 2018;**44**:1482-1488

[78] Jung SI, Seo CH, Jang K, et al. Efficacy of naltrexone in the treatment of chronic refractory itching in burn patients: Preliminary report of an open trial. Journal of Burn Care & Research. 2009;**30**(2):257-260. [discussion: 61]

[79] Hudson DA, Renshaw A. An algorithm for the release of burn contractures of the extremities. Burns. 2006;**32**(6):663-668

Section 3

Negative Pressure Wound Therapy

Chapter 7

Application of Negative Pressure Wound Therapy on Closed Incisions

Chitang J. Joshi, Ji-Cheng Hsieh, Abbas Hassan and Robert D. Galiano

Abstract

Negative pressure wound therapy (NPWT) is widely used for chronic and acute open wounds, with clinically proven benefits of faster wound healing by promoting granulation tissue growth and increased perfusion and facilitating epithelialization and contraction. Improved outcomes on open wounds prompted the application of NPWT on closed surgical incisions. The application of NPWT, in the immediate postoperative period, reduces surgical site infections (SSIs) and wound dehiscence by 50% in high-risk patients. The negative pressure reduces wound edema and improves local perfusion and lymphatic flow, thereby minimizing hematoma and seroma rates. The improved perfusion and oxygenation facilitate quicker wound healing as well as minimize ischemic complications like flap necrosis. Recent literature supports enhanced wound healing and superior scar appearance as well as improved wound maturity, evidenced by 50% more force required to pull apart a sutured incision. Improved outcomes of incisional NPWT are reported from various surgical procedures on abdominal, breast, orthopedic, vascular, cardiac, and plastic surgeries. Further clinical studies and cost-benefit analysis are needed to recommend routine postoperative use of incisional NPWT in high-risk and low-risk patient population.

Keywords: negative pressure wound therapy, incisional NPWT, closed incision NPWT, wound healing, wound dehiscence, surgical site infections

1. Introduction

The concept of negative pressure wound therapy (NPWT) was pioneered in 1997 by Morykwas, applying vacuum-assisted closure (VAC) on a pig wound model. Morykwas' initial methodology involved packing the wound with foam, covering and sealing with an adhesive drape, and applying 125 mm Hg of negative pressure either continuously or intermittently [1]. The rudimentary NPWT led to increased blood flow, granulation tissue, and flap survival, with decreased bacterial growth [1].

NPWT refers to wound healing technology consisting of three major parts: a wound dressing, covers, and a pump [2]. Wound dressing aids in transferring pressure from the pump to the wound itself, and modern NPWT typically utilizes reticulated open-pore polyurethane foam, intended to equalize the negative pressure across the entire wound surface [2]. The cover creates an airtight seal over an open wound, and the pump applies the negative pressure [2, 3].

There are four major types of NPWT [4]. The first is a large, battery-powered NPWT in the acute inpatient setting, while the second is a portable, battery-powered NPWT designed for outpatient use, but cannot be purchased over the counter and tends to be noisy [4]. The third type is a longer-lasting battery-powered NPWT that can be purchased over the counter and is designed to last 7 days and subsequently discarded, while altered models designed for inpatient use that include additional functions, such as negative pressure wound therapy with instillation-dwelling (NPWTi-d) and incisional negative pressure wound therapy (iNPWT), are the last [4].

1.1 Mechanism of action

By drawing fluid out of the wound, negative pressure increases blood flow, decreases the bacterial burden, cleans the wound, reduces local edema, and removes soluble inflammatory mediators that may delay wound healing [2–4]. It has been postulated that NPWT draws antibiotics into the wound, but evidence is lacking [2]. The application of pressure applies forces to the wound, exerting effects macroscopically, through macrodeformation, as well as microscopically, through microdeformation [2, 5]. Naturally, negative pressure on a sealed wound draws the wound edges together [2]. However, it is important to note that the effect is reliant upon tissue parameters such as elasticity and tension, and the strength of the negative pressure does not seem to affect the amount of macrodeformation that occurs [2].

With NPWT, 5–20% of the wound surface experiences tissue stress, and by using a reticulated wound dressing, the action of drawing the wound bed into each pore via negative pressure constitutes the microdeformation that promotes tissue healing processes: increases in cell proliferation, angiogenesis, granulation tissue formation, and epithelialization and decreases in inflammation [2, 5]. NPWT has the potential to grow granulation tissue over exposed bone, tendon, or devices [4]. Specifically, NPWT increases the concentration of VEGF, TGF-beta, FGF-2, PDGF, and IL-8 in the wound, with IL-10 increasing in the body, and decreased concentrations of TNF-alpha, IL-1 beta, and matrix metalloproteases (MMPs) [2]. In patients with type-2 diabetes, the pro-angiogenic and pro-epithelization proteins GDNF family receptor alpha-2 (GFRA2), which complement C1q binding protein (C1QBP), RAB35, and synaptic inositol 1,4,5-triphosphate 5-phosphatase 1 (SYNJ1), were increased [2].

2. NPWT

2.1 Early indications and need for NPWT

Traditional NPWT has been utilized for chronic and acute open wounds and has become a mainstay of wound management [4, 6, 7].

Indications for NPWT are as follows [5, 8]:

- Acute, chronic, and dehisced surgical wounds
- Diabetic, pressure, and venous leg ulcers
- Open abdominal wounds

- Fasciotomies
- Split-thickness skin graft (STSG) recipient sites
- Flaps
- Partial-thickness burns

Contraindications of NPWT include fistulas, malignancy, osteomyelitis, or infection, and NPWT should never be applied over exposed critical anatomic structures or in wounds with necrotic tissue [4, 5]. Despite the benefits of NPWT, there are several key reminders to remember in order for treatment to be effective. The cover and drainage tube must be assessed carefully as loss of seal or fluid buildup in the tube can lead to skin loss or maceration [5]. It is also important to monitor the pump to minimize the risk of exsanguination.

There is significant variability regarding the application of NPWT that depends on wound characteristics [2, 5]. The wound packing can be foam or gauze [2]. The pump may be mechanically or electrically driven [2]. The strength of negative pressure can vary from −50 mm Hg to −150 mm Hg [2]. The pattern of negative pressure application can be intermittent, continuous, or variable, with a continuous pattern the most common [2]. Selection of parameters is typically at the physician's discretion, but a recommended pressure is 125 mm Hg applied in a pattern alternating between a 5-minute negative pressure and a 2-minute suction [4, 5]. Although studies suggest intermittent NPWT is the most effective pattern in inducing granulation tissue formation and increasing blood flow, it also increases pain for the patient [4, 5]. As a result, continuous pressure is often used for painful wounds, as well as wounds with overlying skin grafts, and particularly edematous wounds [5]. Beyond wound outcomes, NPWT reduces the number of dressing changes, healthcare labor, time spent in the hospital, and costs, and this is most demonstrated in portable NPWT, which allows treatment to be done at home [5, 9].

2.2 Current applications

Beyond its indications listed previously, the use of NPWT has been expanding into newer wound types, including tunneling wounds and avascular tissue, and new published case series have demonstrated the use of NPWT in wounds such as necrotizing fasciitis [4, 5, 10]. Alterations to traditional NPWT led to negative wound pressure therapy with installation (NPWT-i) and incisional negative pressure wound therapy (iNPWT), the latter of which is utilized on closed wounds.

3. Incisional NPWT

Incisional NPWT (iNPWT) has been used since 2006, as an adjunct treatment to augment wound healing and prevent surgical site infections (SSI) and wound complications.

3.1 Evolution and development

Surgical incisions are a break in the skin and its defenses in avoiding translocation of infectious pathogens into the deeper tissues. It's imperative to cover and isolate these incisions by a sterile protective dressing in the sterile environment of the operating room. Advances in these sterile protective dressings have taken place over decades and, in the present form, are made up of a nonadherent, antimicrobial-containing dressing covered with sterile gauze or abdominal pads, which are held in place by tapes or transparent film.

In the 1990s, NPWT demonstrated promising results in the management of acute and chronic open wounds, and Argenta and Morykwas proposed improved perfusion and wound contraction, which had a profoundly positive effect on the success of wound healing [1].

Gomoll et al., in 2006, pioneered the idea of incisional NPWT and described the application of NPWT on 35 orthopedic trauma patients, considered high-risk for infections [11]. A permeable nonadherent dressing was applied over the incision and covered with standard VAC sponge cut into 1-inch wide strips and then sealed with conventional VAC adhesive material. The negative pressure was maintained for 3 days, and patients were followed up for SSI for a minimum of 3 weeks. None of these 35 patients reported infections, which led to heightened interest in application of NPWT for surgical incisions.

3.2 Mechanism of action

Efficacy of NPWT depends on a number of factors, namely, foam width, foam thickness, magnitude of negative pressure, and its duration and frequency.

To achieve reproducible and standardized results, the NPWT dressing includes a skin interface layer, which is directly placed over the incision site, over which reticulated foam dressing is secured with occlusive drape. The VAC pump along with the canister is then connected via tubes attached through the foam dressing and secured underneath the occlusive drape to maintain an airtight seal. It's imperative to secure and maintain an airtight seal, in order to achieve efficacy and prevent complications like maceration of peri-wound skin.

Several studies and trials have proposed these mechanisms of iNPWT (**Figure 1**):

- Physical barrier to external contamination
- Microdeformation of the wound edges and release of local growth factors
- Approximation of wound edges and minimizing lateral tension and dead space
- Fluid egress and exudate removal

The negative pressure is commonly used *continuously* within a range of *–75 mm of Hg to –125 mm of Hg*. Although a faster rate of granulation is seen with interrupted pressure, the associated drastic changes in the foam contraction and expansion often render it more painful and impractical for use.

Another alternative, to bridge the gap between continuous and interrupted pressure, is *variable pressure*. It combines the benefit of interrupted pressure and faster granulation tissue growth with gradual and smaller deviations in pressure, in an attempt to minimize pain.

The role of foam width and thickness is important, as it's proportional to the lateral tension attenuation, as described later in the chapter. Hence, a standard foam width of 60 mm is recommended. Cutting thin strips of the foam and using as a construction dressing are also discouraged, as it limits the efficacy and benefits of the iNPWT.

The optimum negative pressure has been a debatable aspect of NPWT. A lot of research focused on negative pressure of –80 mm Hg with positive results, followed

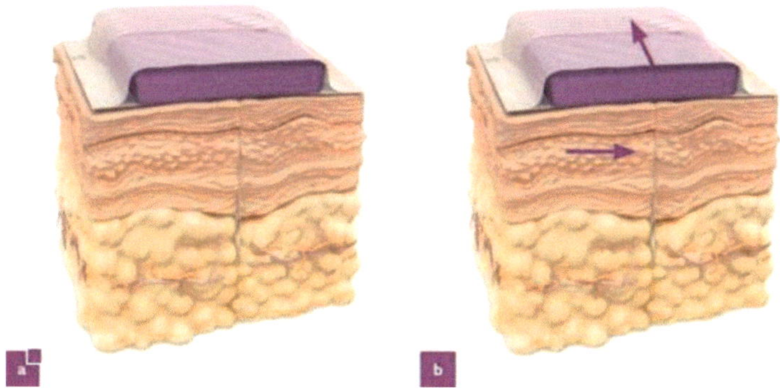

Figure 1.
Cross-sectional depiction of an incision closed with sutures without incisional NPWT (a). Application of incisional NPWT decreases lateral tissue tension and increases incisional apposition (b), reducing dead space. The applied pressure causes microdeformation and release of local growth factors, promoting healing of the surgical incision (reprinted with permission from Ref. [36]).

by a paper published by Morykwas et al., using -125 mm Hg. The results of this trial were promising as it demonstrated improved healing and granulation as compared to the earlier results published by the same team and others. Recent literature and guidelines recommend a pressure of -125 mm Hg; however, pressures ranging from -80, -100, and -125 mm Hg have been employed, and encouraging results have been published.

Application of iNPWT on perineal wounds, following abdominoperineal resection (APR) for colonic and anal lesions, demonstrated improved wound healing and reduced complications and infection rates, while using pressure of -80 mm Hg. The increase in negative pressure beyond -125 mm Hg does not demonstrate improved wound outcomes, either in open or closed wounds.

As the uses and application of the NPWT system develop for closed incision surgical wounds, results of various large-scale clinical trials would emerge, and further modifications would evolve to maximize the clinical benefits of this promising therapeutic modality for postoperative surgical wounds.

3.3 Advantages of iNPWT

Several studies have described the benefits of incisional NPWT (iNPWT) in general, colorectal, cardiac, vascular, plastic, and orthopedic surgeries. These benefits have been classified as immediate, intermediate, and long-term effects and result from the sterile isolation of the incision; mechanical stabilization and reduction in the tensile forces; obliteration of dead space; reduction of local edema, hematoma, and seroma; and increased perfusion and lymphatic flow.

Nam et al. proposed benefits of iNPWT [12], as

- Immediate effects
    - Protection of incision from external contamination
    - Decreased lateral tension on the incision
    - Increased appositional strength
    - Normalized stress distribution

- Increased skin perfusion
- Intermediate effects
  - Decreased edema
  - Decreased hematoma/seroma formation
  - Increased lymphatic flow
- Long-term effects
  - Improved Incision quality
  - Mechanical strength
  - Histology
  - Gene expression

3.3.1 Prevention of external contamination and surgical site infections

Surgical site infections (SSIs) result in significant morbidity and increased healthcare costs, accounting for 21.8% of the 721,800 healthcare-associated infections recorded annually in the United States [13].

SSIs are estimated to increase average hospital stay by 9.6 days, resulting in an added cost of $38,656 and around $10 billion in direct and indirect costs annually [14].

With emphasis on lowering healthcare costs and advancing quality of care, SSIs pose a major physical, psychological, and economic burden.

Incisional NPWT immediately provides protection and isolation of the incision from external contamination. Multiple studies in trauma surgery, general surgery, and plastic surgery have attributed decreased local edema, fluid egress, lower hematoma/seroma rates, lower time to healing, and improved genomic profile, in terms of reduction of pro-inflammatory cytokines and chemokines in surgical incisions covered with NPWT. An international expert panel in 2017 recommended ciNPWT for patients at high risk for surgical site complications [15]. Notable high-risk features include diabetes, ASA score ≥ 3, obesity (BMI ≥ 30 kg/m^2), tobacco use, hypoalbuminemia, corticosteroid use, high-tension wounds and revision surgery.

Multiple studies across different specialties reported a threefold to fivefold reduction in the surgical site infection risk, following the use of ciNPWT [16–18].

Notably, Grauhan and team reported findings of a prospective study of 150 obese patients who underwent cardiac surgery via a median sternotomy. A significant reduction of fourfold in the incidence of wound infection was seen in the iNPWT group compared to conventional dressings, at 1 week of surgery [19]. Similar findings were reported by Matatov in groin infections covered with iNPWT, after vascular procedures (6 vs. 30%, $p = 0.0011$) [20]. Bonds described a reduction in the rate of SSIs in the iNPWT group, after open colectomy (12.5 vs. 29.3%, $p < 0.05$) [21].

Contrastingly, a study analyzing 398 patients concluded incisional NPWT improved short-term wound complications but had no effect on long-term infection rate following knee and hip arthroplasty. A higher proportion of iNPWT patients reported wound drainage at day 7, though similar increase was not seen at different time intervals. This study is the largest RCT comparing outcomes of NPWT dressing in elective lower extremity arthroplasty and supporting improved soft tissue healing response and lower wound-related complications, but no effect on the risk of late superficial or deep infections [22].

Evidence supporting the use of iNPWT in hand and spine surgery is new and fewer. SSIs occur is 0.4–20% of patients undergoing spine surgery and contribute to increased morbidity, hospitalization, and costs [23–26]. Various treatment modalities such as drains, copious irrigation, and prophylactic antibiotics are employed. Adogwa et al. reported a 30% reduction in wound infection rate and 50% reduction in wound dehiscence rates in patients after long-segment thoracolumbar spine fusion and suggested ciNPWT as a safe and effective means of wound management for high-risk spine incisions.

Recent literature suggests incisional NPWT as a safe and effective method in preventing SSIs and wound complications in high-risk patients.

3.3.2 Cost analysis of iNPWT

As modern healthcare strives to deliver quality and efficient yet cost-effective care, continued efforts are warranted to evaluate economic viability of NPWT use and its application in various specialties.

An estimated cost of $100 per day was associated with the use of the PREVENA (V.A.C therapy, KCI, San Antonio, TX) system, which showed significant reduction in SSI risk [27]. With a typical use of 5–7 days, cost of ciNPWT is estimated around $500–700. When used in high-risk populations and higher-cost wound management modality, such additional costs of the NPWT system are validated, as they lead to overall reduction in total healthcare expenditure. SSIs prolong hospital stay, on an average of 9 days, and are associated with an increase in costs up to $20,000 [28].

When compared with indirect costs associated with treatment of wound dehiscence and complications, and direct costs such as daily dressing changes, the economic viability of the iNPWT system in high-risk population seems justified. Chopra et al. found an estimated cost saving of $1456 with ciNPWT use in abdominal wall surgeries. Raymund Horch and his team proposed a cost saving of $163 in obese patients and $203 in morbidly obese patients employing iNPWT in post-bariatric patients undergoing abdominal and thigh dermolipectomy. The authors determined that a 28 and 25% reduction in SSIs' rate in the obese and morbidly obese patients, respectively, was needed to achieve cost savings with iNPWT. Lewis et al. proposed cost savings with iNPWT if wound complications are reduced by one-third in patients undergoing laparotomy for gynecological malignancies [29]. Further evaluation of the applicability of the NPWT system and its costs is warranted in diverse patient population (high vs. low risk), healthcare setups (inpatient vs. at-home), and specialties.

3.3.3 Wound healing

NPWT has been applied successfully as a therapeutic modality to treat open wounds for decades, which led to heightened interest in the scientific community to use it over closed wounds, incisions, and skin grafts. Many trials and studies have proposed the following mechanisms of incisional NPWT:

- Foam dressing protects wound from external mechanical stress.

- Decrease wound tension and tensile forces in deeper dermal layers.

- Continuous removal of exudate and fluids.
- Decrease local edema improving physiologic adaptation of the wound.
- Increase in local perfusion, oxygenation, and lymphatic flow.
- Decrease hematoma/seroma rates.
- Decrease in time-to-heal duration.

On a molecular level, iNPWT has been hypothesized to remove toxic inflammatory mediators and increase the concentration of local tissue growth factors, via microdeformation [30].

An immediate benefit of the iNPWT is the foam dressing that protects the incision/wound from external contamination as well as its ability to minimize the lateral tension around the suture line by 50%. It also normalizes tensile forces in the deep dermal tissue to decrease dead space, which aids in wound healing and reduced seroma/hematoma rates. In wound mechanics, study conducted on an incision made on silicon surface found when iNPWT was applied, 51% more force was required to pull apart a sutured incision, and 43% more force was required to pull apart a stapled incision than non-iNPWT-treated incisions. An interesting correlation was the proportional association between the width of the foam dressing and the force required to pull the incision apart. The study concluded that a foam width of 60 mm is required to increase the tensile strength of the incision.

Studies on earlier techniques of NPWT discouraged the construction method (dressing of the incision by cutting foam into thin strips) as it likely decreased the positive effect of reduced lateral tension on the incision [1].

Early application of iNPWT on pig wound model demonstrated improved healing in terms of mechanical, histomorphometric, and gene expression properties. These incisions showed significantly improved mechanical properties (strain energy density, peak strain) and a narrower scar, extending in the deep dermis [31].

Long-term genomic analysis on surgical wounds reveals pro-inflammatory chemokine and cytokine signals in conventional dressing (sterile absorbent abdominal dressing)-treated incisions compared to iNPWT-treated incisions. Thus, the latter seemed superior in wound strength and wound maturity compared to conventional dressing-covered incisions [31].

Early application of iNPWT promotes fluid egress and continuous removal of exudates. This leads to reduction in local edema, reduced hematoma/seroma rates, improved time to hematoma resolution, decreased time to wound healing, and with split-thickness skin grafts (STSG), improved survival with NPWT [12]. When used with grafts and skin substitutes, the fluid egress with iNPWT minimizes sheer stress and provides tight apposition to the underlying recipient wound bed, which promotes incorporation of the graft or skin substitutes and reepithelialization of graft interstices [32–34]. Maruccia et al. described faster healing, fewer dressing changes, and quicker maturity of mesh skin grafts when combined with NPWT. This combined treatment provides higher integration, better immobilization of the graft, expulsion of fluids, and a moist clean wound bed [35].

The reduction in local edema and removal of fluids in sites such as the abdomen and breast help in reducing the need for postoperative drainage. There is renewed interest in analyzing results to conclude reduced need and duration for postoperative drains. Several studies in general surgery, plastic surgery, and orthopedic surgery have demonstrated reduced drainage with iNPWT-covered incisions. Raymund Horch and his team, in 2014, demonstrated the benefits of iNPWT in a post-bariatric patient population undergoing dermolipectomy of the abdomen and who presented with reduced exudate formation, earlier drain removal, and decreased length of hospitalization [36].

3.3.4 Pain relief

Pain relief with iNPWT has been reported rarely, as very few studies have focused on reporting pain scores with this modality. Maruccia et al., in 2016, reported a statistically significant reduction in pain scores and wound area in skin graft patients. This could be explained by faster healing and improved uptake of the graft, along with less frequent need for dressing changes [35].

3.3.5 Scar appearance

Recent literature shows *scar appearance* improvement with the iNPWT system, across various incision sites. Keeney et al., in 2018, reported a trend toward better outcomes and improved scar appearance in total knee arthroplasty (TKA) patients [22]. Similar improvements have been reported with breast, abdominal, and lower and upper extremity incisions too. This is explained by faster wound healing, decreased time-to-heal time, reduced wound area and lateral tension, and reduced scarring in the deep dermal layers. Optimization in wound healing and avoidance of complications, such as wound dehiscence and hematoma/seroma formation, reduce secondary scarring and augurs well for improved scar appearance.

3.3.6 Perfusion and oxygen saturation

An important aspect of iNPWT is its ability to alter *microcirculation and improve tissue perfusion and oxygen saturation,* in the immediate, intermediate, and long-term analysis of surgical wounds. The purported mechanisms of action are microdeformation of wound and increased neo-angiogenesis via release of local growth factors [37]. Improved perfusion is demonstrated in the cutaneous arterioles (along the skin edges) as well as the deeper tissues, as evidenced by Atkins et al., in peri-sternal perfusion after cardiac surgery via median sternotomy. The iNPWT was also able to compensate for the reduced perfusion rendered by mammary artery harvesting in these patients. In a study published in 2014, Raymund Horch and his team demonstrated improved SaO_2 and blood flow at all time intervals, over abdomen and thigh wounds in post-bariatric surgery patients undergoing dermolipectomy. This was recorded by placing sensors and O_2C probe over the abdominal skin and thighs [36].

Timmers et al. found a fivefold increase in perfusion, assessed with Doppler probes, after application of NPWT over the forearms of healthy volunteers [38].

In a study on iNPWT published in 2016 from the University of Chicago, comprising of 228 patients undergoing immediate expander-based breast reconstruction (study and control groups of 45 and 183, respectively), it was concluded that the application of iNPWT significantly decreased the rate of major mastectomy flap necrosis rate (requiring operative intervention), overall mastectomy flap necrosis rates, and overall complication rates [39].

3.3.7 Lymphatic flow

An important supplement to the improved perfusion is *increased lymphatic flow* around the incision. Lymphatic flow increments aid in reducing hematoma and seroma rates, which are estimated to be reduced by 50–63% with the use of iNPWT. The importance of increased lymphatic flow on reducing seroma/hematoma rates is evidenced by the porcine model study described by Kilpadi and Cunningham, in which significant reduction of hematoma and seroma occurs without fluid collection in the canister [40].

Kilpadi and Cunningham reported 63% reduced hematoma/seroma rates with iNPWT and injected isotope-labeled nanospheres in the subcutaneous tissue to discover their highest concentration in lymph nodes closest to, draining the incision site [40]. Recent literature is overwhelmingly in favor of reduced seroma/hematoma rates, across various surgical procedures covering different surgical specialties and incision sites. To name a few, iNPWT and reduced seroma/hematoma have been demonstrated at flap donor sites, like scapular and latissimus dorsi free flap harvest sites, total hip and knee arthroplasty, over abdominal (e.g., cesarean, laparotomy, and abdominoplasty), thoracic incisions (e.g., sternotomy), breast incisions (expander-based and autologous reconstruction), lower extremity (trauma and fractures), and groin incisions (vascular procedures involving femoral vessels) [40–43].

3.3.8 Hospital stay

Reduced hospital stay with iNPWT use has been demonstrated extensively, via reduced time-to-heal duration, as well as decreased SSI and wound dehiscence and complication rates. A recent systematic review on abdomen procedures estimates reduction of ICU stay but required more extensive clinical RCT and research [44]. Though, it's difficult to quantify this reduction in hospital stay across various procedures, NPWT as an incision management tool has been demonstrated to optimize and accentuate the wound healing process.

3.3.9 Readmission and reoperation rates

These rates have been assessed in a recent meta-analysis comparing efficacy of NPWT in high-risk patients undergoing abdominal wall reconstruction. Both outcomes were low in the iNPWT group as compared to control [9 vs. 14% and 3 vs. 14%, respectively; RR = 0.68 CI (0.46–0.99)].

3.3.10 Wound dehiscence and complication

Wound dehiscence and complications are lowered with the use of iNPWT and its aforementioned benefits. Recent literature estimates a reduction of ~50% reduction in wound dehiscence rates, across various surgical specialties [23, 45–50].

The proposed mechanism of improved wound healing, increased perfusion, decreased infection rates, decreased hematoma/seroma rates, decreased lateral and deep wound tension, improved wound maturity, and strength and obliteration of dead space augurs well for low wound dehiscence and complication rate.

Besides the cost-benefit analysis, an incision management tool with these benefits and improved scar appearance definitely requires further clinical trials and recommendations for use, especially in high-risk patients.

3.4 Complications and risks of iNPWT

Interest in the use of iNPWT has been peaking in the last few years as favorable outcomes seem promising and with easy adaptability and application of at-home single-use canister-based NPWT. This single-use NPWT can be used for

7 days and improves patient acceptability and compliance. A lot of research has been invested in the safety of these systems and to identify complications impeding its widespread use.

The risk of hemorrhage, especially in patients on anticoagulants and with clotting disorders, has been described with the use of iNPWT. Any evidence of fistulas or communication to visceral cavities needs further imaging and management before the application of negative pressure. Allergic reaction to the dressings is a contraindication to the use of iNPWT. Minor skin irritation and ecchymosis are the most frequently encountered complications.

4. Clinical applications of incisional NPWT

The earliest description of the use of negative pressure in wound healing was in the management of soft tissue injury associated with open fractures. The beneficial outcomes seen in various animal models spurred the development of a wide range of clinical indications including abdominal, breast, orthopedic, vascular, cardiac, and plastic surgeries (e.g., skin graft, burns, muscle flap) [51].

4.1 Abdominal wounds

The use of incisional NPWT in high-risk patients undergoing abdominal surgeries decreased wound complications such as surgical site infections and wound healing complications. The primary goals of incisional NPWT wound management include active removal of exudates, estimation of third-space fluid loss, and avoidance of mechanical contamination of the abdominal viscera [51].

With the help of the dressing, NPWT applies negative pressure uniformly, thus promoting healing by reducing edema, approximating the wound, and removing infectious material and exudates [52].

Some studies showed that NPWT improves the removal of abdominal fluid, which helps in early fascial closure. The removal of fluids is especially beneficial in reducing inflammatory responses that may occur [53, 54]. This is supported by the septic/hemorrhagic shock porcine model, which showed that NPWT efficacy was partially due to a reduction in the anti-inflammatory response [55].

On a recent comparative study on incisional NPWT and conventional dressing following abdominal wall reconstruction, the authors demonstrated a statically significant reduction in the incidence of skin dehiscence and overall wound complications in the incisional NPWT group compared with the conventional dressing group [30].

In a study comparing the rates of SSI of patients who underwent surgery for pancreatic, colorectal, or peritoneal surface malignancies between incisional NPWT and conventional dressings, the incidence of SSI was significantly lower in the incisional NPWT group than the conventional group [56].

The use of incisional NPWT as an effective prophylactic tool has been examined in studies from various surgical specialties. The results show that its use facilitates healing of incisional wounds and reduces the incidence of wound healing disorders [57].

4.2 Breast surgery

Breast reconstruction using the expander-/implant-based breast reconstruction is usually performed after mastectomy and plays a crucial role in psychosocial and oncological outcomes in breast cancer patients.

One of the most common and significant complications in the immediate expander-based breast reconstruction is mastectomy flap necrosis, which has been reported to occur in up to 30% of the patients [58]. Authors of a recent study evaluated the incidence of mastectomy flap necrosis in patients with incisional NPWT after immediate expander-based breast reconstruction compared with the incidence in patients with conventional dressing.

The incisional NPWT group had a lower overall complication rate, overall mastectomy flap necrosis rate, and major mastectomy flap necrosis than the conventional dressing group [59].

Besides oncological breast surgery, the use of incisional NPWT was also assessed in a multicenter study on reduction mammoplasty. The results have shown that incisional NPWT applied to closed incision appeared to be most effective on dehiscence in the higher BMI categories and benefit most in preventing complications in the higher tissue resection weight categories [60] (**Figure 2**). The results thus suggest applying incisional NPWT devices in reduction mammoplasty where the BMI is over 25 or resection weight is above 500 mg [60] (**Figure 3**).

The safety and efficacy of incisional NPWT in elderly patients undergoing breast surgery were studied previously. The results of the study suggest that the rates of infections and surgical site events (SSE) were lower with the use of incisional NPWT. The use of incisional NPWT is thus highly recommended in elderly patients, who have significant increased risk of developing SSE when compared with younger patients [61]. Other studies have concluded that incisional NPWT applied to closed surgical incisions on healthy patients after breast reduction surgery prevented postsurgical wound complications significantly [62].

4.3 Orthopedics

Complications related to high-risk lower extremity fractures such as calcaneal, pilon, and tibial plateau are particularly common. Common complications include infection and wound healing problems. In a prospective randomized multicenter clinical trial evaluating the use of NPWT after calcaneus, pilon, or tibial fractures, the authors have found a significant reduction of infection in the NPWT group [48]. The beneficial effects of NPWT on wounds after total ankle replacement or calcaneus fractures were recognized in a study that showed decreased total time required to achieve complete healing, decreased risk of infections, and decreased pain and swelling [63]. Several retrospective studies showed positive effects of incisional NPWT on wounds after open reduction and internal fixation of acetabular fractures. The NPWT group showed reduced rates of wound dehiscence, deep wound infections, and infection rates [64, 65].

A prospective randomized clinical study examined the wounds of patients after total hip arthroplasty using ultrasound examination to evaluate for the development of potential seroma, a possible risk factor for wound infections. The study showed a significant reduction in the seroma size when compared to standard wound dressing and positive effects on wound healing and complication rate [42].

4.4 Cardiac surgery

Despite the use of prophylactic antibiotics, the increasing incidence of postoperative sternal wound infections continues to be a serious problem after surgical cardiac procedures. Sternal wound infections are associated with additional expenses, increased length of stay in the hospital, increased mortality during the first year, and a significant reduction in quality of life [66].

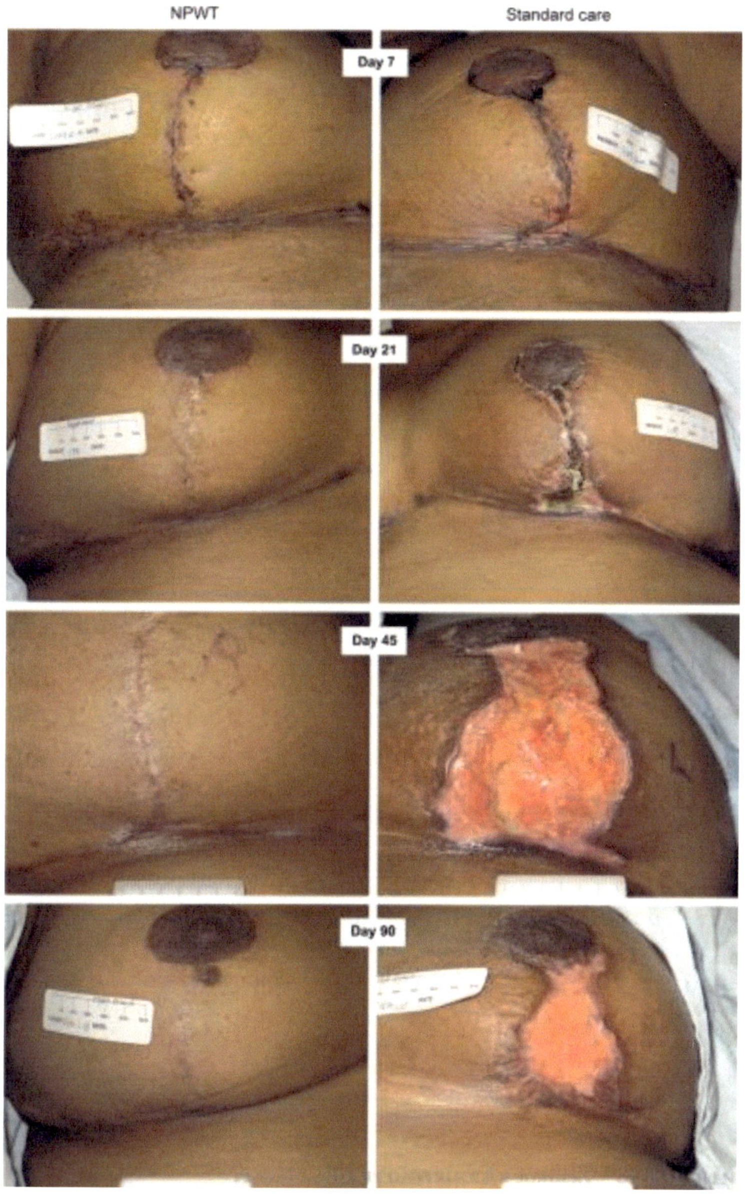

Figure 2.
Progression of incisions in patient treated with iNPWT and standard wound care after bilateral reduction mammaplasty. Wound complications and dehiscence are reduced with iNPWT (reprinted with permission from Ref. [60]).

Risk factors that increase the risk of sternal wound infections include smoking, diabetes, increasing number of grafts, peripheral vascular disease, chronic pulmonary disease, obesity, increased duration of mechanical ventilation, preoperative malnutrition, and harvesting of bilateral internal mammary arteries [67].

The use of incisional NPWT on sternal surgical incisions in patients with multiple comorbidities and consequently a high risk for wound complications was evaluated. Results have shown no wound complications in this high-risk group of patients at least 30 days after surgery and complete wound and surrounding skin healing with the absence of skin lesion due to negative pressure after removal of the dressing [68]. Results from another study also concluded that applying incisional

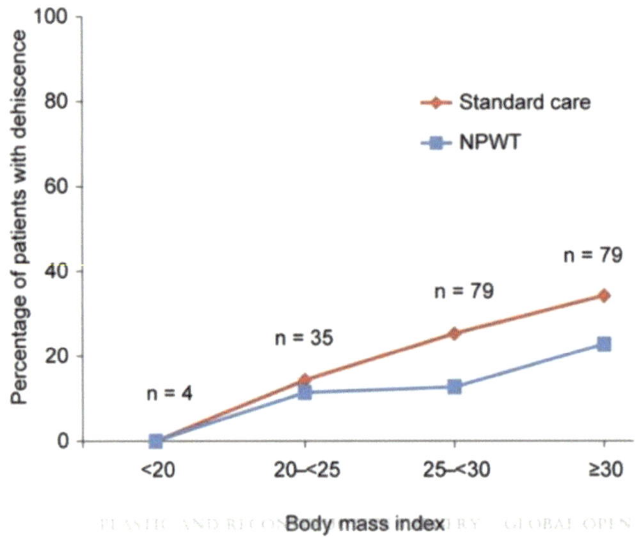

Figure 3.
Relation of body mass index (BMI) on wound dehiscence rates in patients undergoing reduction mammaplasty. The NPWT group shows lower wound dehiscence rates than standard wound care (reprinted with permission from Ref. [60]).

NPWT over clean, closed incisions for the first 6–7 postoperative days reduced the likelihood of postoperative wound infections after median sternotomy not only in high-risk patients but also in a comprehensive patient population [45].

4.5 Vascular surgery

Vascular surgical site infections (SSI) occur as a result of perioperative events that lead to the colonization of the wound and underlying graft with bacterial species. Patients undergoing vascular procedures are at an increased risk of developing an SSI of up to 5% of clean procedures and 30% of clean-contaminated procedures [69]. Severe complications that arise after vascular surgery including leg amputation and death prompted the use of incisional NPWT postoperatively to prevent complications associated with such surgeries. Results of different studies have shown a potential reduction in wound complications and no observed increase in hemorrhage in high-risk patients with severe comorbidities undergoing vascular surgeries [70].

Recent retrospective study on lower leg fasciotomy supports faster wound closure and daily wound size reduction, fewer dressing changes, and shorter hospital stay with NPWT. These factors contribute to significant reduction in surgical site infections, from 30 per cent with standard wound care to 6 per cent with closed incisional NPWT [71].

4.6 Plastic surgery

In plastic surgery, the use of NPWT is particularly important in patients who experienced complications associated with skin graft rejection and its associated partial necrosis. It's also used after excision of large scalp flaps due to injuries and lack of opportunities to cover it with the patient's own skin. NPWT resulted in faster healing and granulation of wounds and a reduction of the overall size [72]. The use of NPWT in large wound surfaces with large amounts of mucus, observed in skin burns, resulted in a significant acceleration in the time taken for patients' healing and rehabilitation. Additional outcomes included wounds that healed better, fewer infection rates, and more elastic tissue preservation [73]. Results from a multicenter, prospective randomized controlled, within-patient study involving our center and senior author (RDG) provided high-level evidence supporting significantly reduced wound complications following application of iNPWT in susceptible patients [60].

5. Conclusion

Advances in surgical and sterilization techniques have largely mitigated risk of wound complications and SSI rates; however, these complications till date pose a major physical, financial, and psychological challenge in the postoperative phase of treatment. Incisional NPWT presents a promising treatment modality for surgical wounds and incisions, with its proposed benefits in reducing infections, preventing wound dehiscence and optimizing wound healing and scarring. Randomized controlled trials and further clinical research are warranted to develop guidelines to the safe, effective, and routine use of iNPWT. However, in the present economic model of healthcare, efficacy of a treatment modality alone does not justify its use, and a large-scale cost-benefit analysis is warranted to rationalize its use in high-risk and low-risk postoperative patients.

Acknowledgements

The authors would like to thank Abbas Hassan, Rou Wan, and Dr. Jing Liu for their valuable inputs and contribution.

Conflict of interest

The authors declare no conflict of interest.

Notes/thanks

The first author CJJ would like to immensely thank senior author RDG for his unending support, guidance, and inspiration to strive to be perfect.

Author details

Chitang J. Joshi, Ji-Cheng Hsieh, Abbas Hassan and Robert D. Galiano*
Department of Plastic and Reconstructive Surgery, Feinberg School of Medicine, Northwestern University, Chicago, IL, United States

*Address all correspondence to: rgaliano@nm.org

References

[1] Argenta LC, Morykwas MJ. Vacuum-assisted closure: A new method for wound control and treatment. Clinical experience. Annals of Plastic Surgery. 1997;**38**(6):563-576

[2] Borys S, Ludwig-Slomczynska AH, Seweryn M, et al. Negative pressure wound therapy in the treatment of diabetic foot ulcers may be mediated through differential gene expression. Acta Diabetologica. 2019;**56**(1):115-120. DOI: 10.1007/s00592-018-1223-y

[3] Condé-Green A, Chung TWL, Holton LH, Hui-Chou HG, Zhu Y, Wang HD, et al. Incisional negative-pressure wound therapy versus conventional dressings following abdominal wall reconstruction: A comparative study. Annals of Plastic Surgery. 2013;**71**(4):394-397

[4] Jaffe L, Wu SC. Dressings, topical therapy, and negative pressure wound therapy. Clinics in Podiatric Medicine and Surgery. 2019;**36**:397-411. DOI: 10.1016/j.cpm.2019.02.005

[5] Rosenbaum AJ, Banerjee S, Rezak KM, Uhl RL. Advances in wound management. Journal of the American Academy of Orthopaedic Surgeons. 2018;**26**(23):833-843

[6] Sahebally SM, McKevitt K, Stephens I, et al. Negative pressure wound therapy for closed laparotomy incisions in general and colorectal surgery: A systematic review and meta-analysis. JAMA Surgery. 2018;**153**(11):e183467

[7] Javed AA, Teinor J, Wright M, et al. Negative pressure wound therapy for surgical-site infections: A randomized trial. Annals of Surgery. 2018;**269**(6):1034-1040

[8] Yao M, Fabbi M, Hayashi H, et al. A retrospective cohort study evaluating efficacy in high-risk patients with chronic lower extremity ulcers treated with negative pressure wound therapy. International Wound Journal. 2014;**11**(5):483-488

[9] Shine J, Efanov JI, Paek L, Coeugniet É, Danino MA, Izadpanah A. Negative pressure wound therapy as a definitive treatment for upper extremity wound defects: A systematic review. International Wound Journal. 2019;**16**(4):960-967. DOI: 10.1111/iwj.13128

[10] Reider K, McElroy E, Lemay S. The use of negative pressure with instillation and dwell for the treatment of necrotizing fasciitis. Cureus. 2018;**10**(10):e3515. DOI: 10.7759/cureus.3515

[11] Gomoll AH, Lin A, Harris MB. Incisional vacuum-assisted closure therapy. Journal of Orthopaedic Trauma. 2006;**20**(10):705-709

[12] Nam D, Sershon RA, Levine BR, Della Valle CJ. The use of closed incision negative-pressure wound therapy in orthopaedic surgery. Journal of the American Academy of Orthopaedic Surgeons. 2018;**26**(9):295-302

[13] Magill SS, Edwards JR, Bamberg W, et al. Emerging infections program healthcare-associated infections and antimicrobial use prevalence survey team: Multistate point-prevalence survey of health care-associated infections. The New England Journal of Medicine. 2014;**370**(13):1198-1208

[14] Shepard J, Ward W, Milstone A, et al. 16. Financial impact of surgical site infections on hospitals: The hospital management perspective. JAMA Surgery. 2013;**148**(10):907-914

[15] Willy C, Agarwal A, Andersen CA, et al. Closed incision negative pressure therapy: International multidisciplinary consensus recommendations.

International Wound Journal. 2017;**14**(2):385-398

[16] Cooper HJ, Bas MA. Closed-incision negative-pressure therapy versus anti-microbial dressings after revision hip and knee surgery: A comparative study. The Journal of Arthroplasty. 2016;**31**:1047e52

[17] Karlakki SL, Hamad AK, Whittall C, Graham NM, Banerjee RD, Kuiper JH. Incisional negative pressure wound therapy dressings (iNPWTd) in routine primary hip and knee arthroplasties: A randomised controlled trial. Bone & Joint Research. 2016;**5**:328e37

[18] Redfern RE, Cameron-Ruetz C, O'Drobinak SK, Chen JT, Beer KJ. Closed incision negative pressure therapy effects on postoperative infection and surgical site complication after total hip and knee arthroplasty. The Journal of Arthroplasty. 2017;**32**:3333e9

[19] GrauhanO,NavasardyanA,HofmannM, Müller P, Stein J, Hetzer R. Prevention of poststernotomy wound infections in obese patients by negative pressure wound therapy. The Journal of Thoracic and Cardiovascular Surgery. 2013;**145**(5):1387-1392

[20] Matatov T, Reddy KN, Doucet LD, Zhao CX, Zhang WW. Experience with a new negative pressure incision management system in prevention of groin wound infection in vascular surgery patients. Journal of Vascular Surgery. 2013;**57**(3):791-795

[21] Bonds AM, Novick TK, Dietert JB, Araghizadeh FY, Olson CH. Incisional negative pressure wound therapy significantly reduces surgical site infection in open colorectal surgery. Diseases of the Colon and Rectum. 2013;**56**(12):1403-1408

[22] Keeney JA, Cook JL, Clawson SW, Aggarwal A, Stannard JP. Incisional negative pressure wound therapy devices improve short-term wound complications, but not long-term infection rate following hip and knee arthroplasty. The Journal of Arthroplasty. 2019;**34**:723-728

[23] Adogwa O, Fatemi P, Perez E, et al. Negative pressure wound therapy reduces incidence of postoperative wound infection and dehiscence after long-segment thoracolumbar spinal fusion: A single institutional experience. The Spine Journal. 2014;**14**(12):2911-2917

[24] Ousey KJ, Atkinson RA, Williamson JB, Lui S. Negative pressure wound therapy (NPWT) for spinal wounds: A systematic review. The Spine Journal. 2013;**13**(10):1393-1405

[25] Jones GA, Butler J, Lieberman I, Schlenk R. Negative-pressure wound therapy in the treatment of complex postoperative spinal wound infections: Complications and lessons learned using vacuum-assisted closure. Journal of Neurosurgery. Spine. 2007;**6**(5):407-411

[26] Ploumis A, Mehbod AA, Dressel TD, Dykes DC, Transfeldt EE, Lonstein JE. Therapy of spinal wound infections using vacuum-assisted wound closure: Risk factors leading to resistance to treatment. Journal of Spinal Disorders & Techniques. 2008;**21**(5):320-323

[27] Kim JJ, Franczyk M, Gottlieb LJ, Song DH. Cost-effective alternative for negative-pressure wound therapy. Plastic and Reconstructive Surgery. Global Open. 2017;**5**:e1211

[28] deLissovoyG,FraemanK,HutchinsV, Murphy D, Song D, Vaughn BB. Surgical site infection: Incidence and impact on hospital utilization and treatment costs. American Journal of Infection Control. 2009;**37**:387-397

[29] Lewis LS, Convery PA, Bolac CS, et al. Cost of care using prophylactic

negative pressure wound vacuum on closed laparotomy incisions. Gynecologic Oncology. 2014;**132**(3):684-689

[30] Tran BN, Johnson AR, Shen C, Lee BT, Lee ES. Closed-incision negative-pressure therapy efficacy in abdominal wall reconstruction in high-risk patients: A meta-analysis. The Journal of Surgical Research. 2019;**241**:63-71

[31] Kilpadi DV, Lessing C, Derrick K. Healed porcine incisions previously treated with a surgical incision management system: Mechanical, histomorphometric, and gene expression properties. Aesthetic Plastic Surgery. 2014;**38**(4):767-778

[32] Dadaci M, Isci ET, Ince B, et al. Negative pressure wound therapy in the early period after hand and forearm replantation: Is it safe? Journal of Wound Care. 2016;**25**(6):350-355

[33] Lesiak AC, Shafritz AB. Negative-pressure wound therapy. The Journal of Hand Surgery. 2013;**38**(9):1828-1832

[34] Watt AJ, Friedrich JB, Huang JI. Advances in treating skin defects of the hand: Skin substitutes and negative-pressure wound therapy. Hand Clinics. 2012;**28**(4):519-528

[35] Maruccia M, Onesti MG, Sorvillo V, Albano A, Dessy LA, Carlesimo B, et al. An alternative treatment strategy for complicated chronic wounds: Negative pressure therapy over mesh skin graft. BioMed Research International. 2017;**2017**:7. DOI: 10.1155/2017/83952

[36] Horch RE. Incisional negative pressure wound therapy for high-risk wounds. Journal of Wound Care. 2015;**24**(4 Suppl):21-28

[37] Orgill DP, Bayer LR. Update on negative-pressure wound therapy. Plastic and Reconstructive Surgery. 2011;**127**(Suppl 1):105S-115S

[38] Timmers MS, Le Cessie S, Banwell P, Jukema GN. The effects of varying degrees of pressure delivered by negative-pressure wound therapy on skin perfusion. Annals of Plastic Surgery. 2005;**55**(6):665-671

[39] Ooi AS, Song DH. Discussion: Does the use of incisional negative-pressure wound therapy prevent mastectomy flap necrosis in immediate expander-based breast reconstruction? Plastic and Reconstructive Surgery. 2016;**138**(3):567-569

[40] Kilpadi DV, Cunningham MR. Evaluation of closed incision management with negative pressure wound therapy (CIM): Hematoma/seroma and involvement of the lymphatic system. Wound Repair and Regeneration. 2011;**19**(5):588-596

[41] Schmedes GW, Banks CA, Malin BT, et al. Massive flap donor sites and the role of negative pressure wound therapy. Otolaryngology and Head and Neck Surgery. 2012;**147**(6):1049-1053

[42] Pachowsky M, Gusinde J, Klein A, et al. Negative pressure wound therapy to prevent seromas and treat surgical incisions after total hip arthroplasty. International Orthopaedics. 2012;**36**(4):719-722

[43] Mark KS, Alger L, Terplan M. Incisional negative pressure therapy to prevent wound complications following cesarean section in morbidly obese women: A pilot study. Surgical Innovation. 2013;**21**(4):345-349

[44] Cirocchi R, Birindelli A, Biffl WL, Mutafchiyski V, Popivanov G, Chiara O, et al. What is the effectiveness of the negative pressure wound therapy (NPWT) in patients treated with open abdomen technique? A systematic review and meta-analysis. The Journal

of Trauma and Acute Care Surgery. 2016;**81**(3):575-584

[45] Grauhan O, Navasardyan A, Tutkun B, Hennig F, Müller P, Hummel M, et al. Effect of surgical incision management on wound infections in a poststernotomy patient population. International Wound Journal. 2014;**11**(Suppl. 1):6-9

[46] Dohmen PM, Misfeld M, Borger MA, Mohr FW. Closed incision management with negative pressure wound therapy. Expert Review of Medical Devices. 2014;**11**(4):395-402

[47] Karlakki S, Brem M, Giannini S, et al. Negative pressure wound therapy for management of the surgical incision in orthopaedic surgery: A review of evidence and mechanisms for an emerging indication. Bone & Joint Research. 2013;**2**(12):276-284

[48] Stannard JP, Volgas DA, McGwin G 3rd, et al. Incisional negative pressure wound therapy after high-risk lower extremity fractures. Journal of Orthopaedic Trauma. 2012;**26**(1):37-42

[49] Stannard JP, Gabriel A, Lehner B. Use of negative pressure wound therapy over clean, closed surgical incisions. International Wound Journal. 2012;**9**(Suppl. 1):32-39

[50] Atkins BZ, Wooten MK, Kistler J, et al. Does negative pressure wound therapy have a role in preventing poststernotomy wound complications? Surgical Innovation. 2009;**16**(2):140-146

[51] Bovill E, Banwell PE, Teot L, Eriksson E, Song C, Mahoney J, et al. Topical negative pressure wound therapy: A review of its role and guidelines for its use in the management of acute wounds. International Wound Journal. 2008;**5**(4):511-529

[52] Lindstedt S, Malmsjö M, Hansson J, Hlebowicz J, Ingemansson R. Pressure transduction and fluid evacuation during conventional negative pressure wound therapy of the open abdomen and NPWT using a protective disc over the intestines. BMC Surgery. 2012;**12**(1):4

[53] Kaplan M, Banwell P, Orgill DP, Ivatury RR, Demetriades D, Moore FA, et al. Guidelines for the management of the open abdomen. Wounds-A Compendium of Clinical Research and Practice. 2005;**17**:1-24

[54] Franklin ME, Alvarez A, Russek K. Negative pressure therapy: A viable option for general surgical management of the open abdomen. Surgical Innovation. 2012;**19**(4):353-363

[55] Kubiak BD, Albert SP, Gatto LA, Snyder KP, Maier KG, Vieau CJ, et al. Peritoneal negative pressure therapy prevents multiple organ injury in a chronic porcine sepsis and ischemia/reperfusion model. Shock. 2010;**34**(5):525-534

[56] Blackham AU, Farrah JP, McCoy TP, Schmidt BS, Shen P. Prevention of surgical site infections in high-risk patients with laparotomy incisions using negative-pressure therapy. The American Journal of Surgery. 2013;**205**(6):647-654

[57] Wiegering A, Dietz UA, Corteville C, Plaßmeier L, Jurowich C, Germer CT, et al. Impact of incisional negative pressure wound therapy on perineal wound healing after abdominoperineal rectum extirpation. International Journal of Colorectal Disease. 2017;**32**(2):291-293

[58] Moyer HR, Losken A. Predicting mastectomy skin flap necrosis with indocyanine green angiography: The gray area defined. Plastic and Reconstructive Surgery. 2012;**129**(5):1043-1048

[59] Kim DY, Park SJ, Bang SI, Mun GH, Pyon JK. Does the use of incisional negative-pressure wound therapy prevent mastectomy flap necrosis in immediate expander-based breast reconstruction? Plastic and Reconstructive Surgery. 2016;**138**(3):558-566

[60] Galiano RD, Hudson D, Shin J, van der Hulst R, Tanaydin V, Djohan R, et al. Incisional negative pressure wound therapy for prevention of wound healing complications following reduction mammaplasty. Plastic and Reconstructive Surgery—Global Open. 2018;**6**(1):e1560

[61] Pellino G, Sciaudone G, Candilio G, De Fatico GS, Landino I, Della Corte A, et al. Preventive NPWT over closed incisions in general surgery: Does age matter? International Journal of Surgery. 2014;**12**:S64-S68

[62] Tanaydin V, Beugels J, Andriessen A, Sawor JH, Van der Hulst RR. Randomized controlled study comparing disposable negative-pressure wound therapy with standard care in bilateral breast reduction mammoplasty evaluating surgical site complications and scar quality. Aesthetic Plastic Surgery. 2018;**42**(4):927-935

[63] DeCarbo WT, Hyer CF. Negative-pressure wound therapy applied to high-risk surgical incisions. The Journal of Foot and Ankle Surgery. 2010;**49**(3):299-300

[64] Reddix JR, Tyler HK, Kulp B, Webb LX. Incisional vacuum-assisted wound closure in morbidly obese patients undergoing acetabular fracture surgery. American Journal of Orthopedics. 2009;**38**(9):446-449

[65] Reddix JR, Leng XI, Woodall J, Jackson B, Dedmond B, Webb LX. The effect of incisional negative pressure therapy on wound complications after acetabular fracture surgery. Journal of Surgical Orthopaedic Advances. 2010;**19**(2):91-97

[66] Hollenbeak CS, Murphy DM, Koenig S, Woodward RS, Dunagan WC, Fraser VJ. The clinical and economic impact of deep chest surgical site infections following coronary artery bypass graft surgery. Chest. 2000;**118**(2):397-402

[67] Lu JC, Grayson AD, Jha P, Srinivasan AK, Fabri BM. Risk factors for sternal wound infection and mid-term survival following coronary artery bypass surgery. European Journal of Cardio-Thoracic Surgery. 2003;**23**(6):943-949

[68] Colli A. First experience with a new negative pressure incision management system on surgical incisions after cardiac surgery in high risk patients. Journal of Cardiothoracic Surgery. 2011;**6**(1):160

[69] Mangram AJ, Horan TC, Pearson ML, Silver LC, Jarvis WR, Hospital Infection Control Practices Advisory Committee. Guideline for prevention of surgical site infection, 1999. Infection Control and Hospital Epidemiology. 1999;**20**(4):247-280

[70] Weir G. The use of a surgical incision management system on vascular surgery incisions: A pilot study. International Wound Journal. 2014;**11**(s1):10-12

[71] Acosta S, Björck M, Wanhainen A. Negative-pressure wound therapy for prevention and treatment of surgical-site infections after vascular surgery. The British Journal of Surgery. 2017;**104**(2):e75-e84

[72] Gupta S. Optimal use of negative pressure wound therapy for skin grafts. International Wound Journal. 2012;**9**:40-47

[73] Bloemen MC, van der Wal MB, Verhaegen PD, Nieuwenhuis MK, van Baar ME, van Zuijlen PP, et al. Clinical effectiveness of dermal substitution in burns by topical negative pressure: A multicenter randomized controlled trial. Wound Repair and Regeneration. 2012;**20**(6):797-805